Gut Feelings

Gut Feelings

A FASCINATING TRUE STORY OF A FAMILY FIGHTING FOR THE LIFE OF THEIR CHILD WHO LOST HIS GUTS TO ULCERATIVE COLITIS

—

Ahmed Abo Sara
Foreword by Lissa Coffey

We hope that sharing our story can comfort and support those out there who are going through this illness and suffering both physically, emotionally, and spiritually

Printed by

ISBN-1500278963
ISBN-9781500278960
Library of Congress Control Number: 2015909216
CreateSpace Independent Publishing Platform
North Charleston, South Carolina

Dear Reader!

This book is written in two parts:

Part I, is an overview on ulcerative colitis (UC), it describes the disease and its causes, symptoms, methods of diagnosis, and treatment. It also answers common questions and concerns on the disease that UC patients or their caregivers may have.

Part II, is Sam's true story - Gut Feelings.

Table of Contents

Foreword

"IN HIS NEW BOOK, Dr. Abo Sara chronicles the experiences he went through as his son, Sam, struggled with ulcerative colitis from a very young age. We all have challenges in this lifetime. How we rise up to meet these struggles says a lot about our character. When we face these difficulties head on and then continue to help others dealing with the same issues, then we understand the connection between us. There are no coincidences and no accidents. By sharing his story, Dr. Abo Sara offers the knowledge and wisdom that he garnered on his journey to anyone who is traveling on a similar path. It can be incredibly scary and stressful to navigate through any illness. But when a child's life is at a stake, the emotions and complicated decisions that must be made can be too much for anyone to bear. Dr. Abo Sara explains the medical lingo involved, and lays out several treatment options for ulcerative colitis. His genuine concern and thorough research is evident. Readers are along with him and his son every step of the way as they sort through their own difficulties and their way to a positive resolution.

I first met Dr. Abo Sara when I took my cat Suki into his veterinary clinic for a check-up. I was immediately taken with Dr. Abo Sara's kindness and gentle, compassionate nature. Every one of us has a purpose, a dharma, and I could see that Dr. Abo Sara was clearly in his dharma with his medical practice. Suki is generally skittish and neurotic, but in Dr. Abo Sara's presence she was calm and at ease. I knew there was something special about this man if he could win over my crazy cat readily!

For anyone who is looking for guidance in this area, I highly recommend Dr. Abo Sara's book. His help in sorting through the obstacles is invaluable because he's been through it himself. His story is fascinating and inspirational!"

Lissa Coffey is a lifestyle expert, media personality, and the founder of CoffeyTalk.com

Preface

Over one million Americans are believed to be suffering from inflammatory bowel disease. Crohn's disease and ulcerative colitis strike children, teenagers and young adults in the prime of life.

ULCERATIVE COLITIS (UC) IS A chronic inflammation of the colon. The exact cause of UC is unknown and the disease is currently classified as an auto-immune illness, meaning that the immune system is attacking its own body. Classic symptoms of UC include bouts of diarrhea associated with urgency to use the bathroom, blood in stool, and abdominal pain. The disease also causes open sores or ulcerations on the innermost lining of the colon. Most often UC is diagnosed in people between the ages of 15-35, but about 10% of cases occur in younger children.

A few decades ago, people with ulcerative colitis had near zero survival rates. This was because the nature of the disease was unknown and doctors were unsure of how to treat it. Now due to the major discoveries regarding the disease, it is rare to die from UC. Advances in research made this possible. Currently there are many treatment options on the market but unfortunately there is no cure yet. Colon resection is really the only true "cure", and it still doesn't eliminate all of the issues. A lot of the time you are trading one evil for another. However, colon resection will severely decrease the risk of developing colon cancer, a commonly occurring cancer in patients with UC.

New medications are being introduced all the time and are increasingly successful. The use of Cyclosporine and the newest biologic therapies like Remicade have saved many patients with ulcerative colitis from undergoing surgery and losing their colon. For children who, in past decades, would waste away and inevitably die, there are now several options of purified diets given by intravenous injection or by stomach tube feeding. These are easily absorbed in the intestine with virtually no residue coming through. Research on genetics of affected people and diagnostic tests has been met with substantial success. The collaborative research projects by various medical groups and pharmaceutical companies have uncovered fine details of the disease. These advances are giving researchers legitimate reasons for optimism. However, more research is needed to determine what exactly causes UC and how it can be cured or even prevented.

This book was written with the following objectives:

1. By sharing our experience, feelings, and the story of our son who was literally ravaged by UC, we hope that patients suffering from this debilitating disease and their families will find this information useful and provide them with kind comfort and support.
2. Patients and their families can arm themselves with extensive and advanced information on UC clear and easy-to-understand language. They will learn the causes of UC, the triggering foods, how to recognize the warning signs of UC, how to learn about the risks of having UC, how to understand the medical tests and how to diagnose UC.
3. This book will empower patients and their families with up-to-date information on UC and advice on how to make better decisions about the various treatment options. Along the way I will introduce you to my experience with members of the medical teams.
4. Real-life practical tips are listed throughout the book to help both patients and their caregivers on various aspects of the disease; such as how to choose the right doctor for this illness, how to deal with difficult moments at school or at work, how to make traveling easier with UC, how to avoid distress associated with caring for a loved one with this chronic illness, how to make UC therapies affordable, how to deal with social

challenges, how to lower the emotional impact of UC on the patient and their family, how to deal with the potential parental self-guilt, where to seek additional information about the disease, and much more.

In this book we neither promote nor recommend any therapy or treatment. Any material of interest should be discussed with the family physician. This information is not intended to replace the advice of a doctor.

The author disclaims any liability for the decisions you make based on this information.

Introduction

For many years, ulcerative colitis (UC) was a fact of life for our son, Sam. He began showing the disease's debilitating symptoms when he was 2 years and 8 months old. At first, the doctor said "Sam has a stomach flu virus. We see this every day. There is nothing to worry about. He will recover in a couple of days." Soon after we realized that Sam had a serious illness called ulcerative colitis and that its cause was unknown. Sam had several flare ups, many complications, and failed to respond to various medications including steroids and potent immunosuppressive drugs. We took him as far as we could to seek help. We were referred to several specialists and we moved to 4 states in less than 3 years looking for the doctor who could cure our son.

Before this young child reached his 7th birthday, he was hospitalized 26 times, had general anesthesia 23 times, had endoscopic examination of his esophagus, stomach, small and large intestine 21 times, had several abdominal CT scans and radiographs, had two major surgeries averaging 4½ hours each, had 5 blood transfusions, and countless doctor visits. We stayed with him in hospitals for so long that the hospitals almost felt like our home. We even joked with doctors and nurses and asked if we could rent a room in the hospital on a monthly basis. Sam had countless blood drawings for laboratory tests and numerous intravenous sets, central lines, and stomach tubes for fluid therapy and feeding.

Doctors initially tried treating Sam's illness with a variety of steroids and other anti-inflammatory medications, but none had a lasting effect. Sam was on several medications including prednisone, Imuran, cyclosporine, Pentasa, sulfasalazine, antibiotics like Flagyl and ciprofloxacin, and iron supplements all at the same time and for several years. Sam experienced serious side effects of these medications which included, among others, impaired growth both in height and weight, facial and body hair overgrowth, moon face, and mood changes. While he was on these medications he did not grow even an inch in height in 5 years. He also became severely immunosuppressed because of these medications and contracted chickenpox, episodes of high fever, and repeated attacks of colds.

Doctors tried juggling his medications for more than 4 years but by March 30, 2001, they had run out of options. We finally accepted the fact that there would be no resolution to Sam's aggressive illness except surgery. Doctors ended up removing his entire large intestine. He started doing much better soon after surgery. He gained weight, started to grow again, and his quality of his life improved tremendously. But he was not free of post-surgical complications, including loose stool, dehydration and pouchitis (inflammation of the pouch) that lasted for almost 5 years. At the time of writing this book, Sam is 21 years old and seemed to appear healthy and to enjoy life. He has just finished his medical assistant program at a local college and is enjoying his job at a local medical office.

Thinking back, we wish that the first doctor we visited was correct, that my Sam had had a stomach flu virus infection and that there was nothing to worry about, instead of a lifelong series of tragedy. After years of reflection on the disease, we could not find of any apparent genetic link to Sam's colitis. No one on either side of our family has had this problem. Sam's sister is healthy. Nevertheless, we are keeping our fingers crossed. Sam was born healthy by normal delivery and with no complications.

Being his father, I was very attached to my son and extensively involved in his illness. I stayed with him in hospitals all of the time and lived every moment of his pain and suffering. I took a leave of absence from my job after I exhausted all of my accumulated vacation time, personal leaves, medical leaves, holidays, weekends, and any time off that I could obtain.

In spite of my medical background as a veterinarian, navigating his illness was very challenging. It was a shocking experience for a father to have his 2 year old child suffering from a serious illness of unknown cause. At the beginning of his illness, any piece of information we received about his laboratory findings felt like a mental shock and heart- wrenching news. This was particularly true during the first few weeks of trying to reach a diagnosis of his illness and assess the extent of damage in his gut. Our nerves were in a constant status of high alert.

I gathered tremendous information about the disease through searching scientific literature, the internet, the Crohn's and Colitis website, talking to specialists and from my day-to-day experience with my son. I kept extensive daily notes on his symptoms, response to medications, diaries of food he was eating, description of his pain and its level, his activity level, laboratory reports, and recognition of his potential flare up warning signs along with other daily observations.

I decided to write this book about what I went through with the hope that someone could benefit from it. Although extensive details on the disease's nature, causes, diagnosis and treatment are presented in **Chapter One**, this book primarily describes our experience with our son's debilitating illness and is not intended to be an encyclopedia of every aspect of ulcerative colitis nor a review of literature on the disease or a comprehensive study or a guideline on ulcerative colitis. It basically details the everyday challenges that faced this young boy and his family.

It is important to seek medical attention if you think that you or a loved one may be plagued by this disease. Managing symptoms can be more successful when the disease is diagnosed early. Finding an experienced doctor who deals with the disease on daily basis is the key to living with this illness. If your only option ends up being a colon resection, make sure you are familiar with all of the challenges after surgery. Stay positive and never forget the power of prayer.

Financially, in spite of our good health insurance plan, this illness cost us thousands of dollars, especially when treatments were out of state. Some laboratory tests were very expensive and some were not covered by the insurance at all. However, having my son stable and sleeping without pain or bleeding was priceless.

I hope this book helps you in your journey through the challenges presented with UC, whether you or a loved one have it. It is written in plain everyday language. When their use is required, the medical terminologies are clearly explained. It is a good experience for the patients and their caregivers to get used to these medical terminologies because doctors will use them every day in discussing their plans of diagnosis and treatments with family members.

Each chapter in this book is self-explanatory and was written independently of other chapters. You can skip any chapter and read the chapter of your interest first and still get a complete understanding of the desired subject. Extensive notes and recommendations are presented throughout the book on how to deal with the daily challenges of UC and its emotional impact on both the patients and families.

Part I

CHAPTER 1

Ulcerative Colitis -An Overview

What Is Ulcerative Colitis?

Ulcerative Colitis (UC) is a chronic inflammation of the colon. The disease typically starts at the lowest part of the colon, which is the rectum, and gradually progresses through varying lengths of the colon. As the name "ulcerative" implies, the disease causes open sores or ulcers on the innermost lining (mucosa) of the colon.

What Causes Ulcerative Colitis?

The exact cause of UC is unknown. The disease is presently classified as an autoimmune disorder meaning that the immune system is attacking its own body and causing the damage.

How does the immune system normally work? In simple terms, the immune system helps the body fight off potentially harmful germs such as bacteria, viruses, and fungi. In a normal healthy person, when the immune system detects a harmful substance, it gets alarmed and orders a flood of defense cells (inflammatory cells) to gather at the site and to combat the foreign invader. The outcome of this battle is either the immune system wins, kills the invader, and gets rid of it, or the invader wins and causes an illness in our body.

How does the immune system work in patients with ulcerative colitis? In people with UC, it is suspected that the local immune system in their colon is defected and overreacts to an invader "trigger" that normally would not evoke such an exaggerated immune response. In a stretch of imagination, it is just like over-welding two pieces of metal that end up burnt and distorted. Similarly, the immune system in patients with UC over-reacts to a "trigger" which results in severe inflammation in the colon, leading to erosions and ulcerations on its lining. The defense system is essentially attacking its own body.

Why is the immune system acting out of control in ulcerative colitis patients? The cause of the over-activation of the immune system in patients with UC is suspected to be a defect in the immune regulation "switch" within the colon which once "turned on", does not "turn off" at the right time. What causes this defect in the regulator system is unknown.

What turned on the immune system in the first place in ulcerative colitis patients? It is unknown what triggers the "on switch" of the immune system in the first place in patients with UC. It's suspected that the immune system get stimulated by some microorganisms in the gut under some favored environment conditions created by certain food or other environmental factors. Neither the nature of these environmental factors nor the identities of these microorganisms are known, if any at all.

In the USA, ulcerative colitis has been diagnosed with increasing incidence in immigrants of various nationalities. It has been hypothesized that westernization, including excessive sanitary precautions and changes in the diet, to a diet rich in fats and processed foods, may influence the bacterial flora in the digestive system, which in turn triggers the local immune system to initiate the inflammation.

Is ulcerative colitis contagious? Ulcerative colitis is not transmissible from affected to healthy persons and thus it is not contagious. No viruses, bacteria, food allergens, or toxins have been identified to cause UC. However, their involvement as triggering agents of the immune system has not been totally ruled out. Some scientists suspect that UC is caused by germs that have not yet been identified.

Does stress trigger ulcerative colitis? Although stress and anxiety do not cause UC, these factors aggravate symptoms of UC.

Does food trigger ulcerative colitis? Which foods make symptoms of UC worse? There are no specific diets that have been proven to cause UC, to keep it in remission, or to cure it. However, many patients share a particular food that aggravates symptoms of UC, particularly while experiencing a flare up, but it is never the same food for all patients. Some of the more common symptom-worsening foods include beverages like alcohol and carbonated drinks, dairy food like ice cream, milk and cheese, spicy food, caffeine, food with high insoluble fiber like beans, bran, seeds, popcorn, and nuts, raw vegetables and citrus fruits, red meat, sugars, high-fat food like butter, fried and greasy food served at fast food restaurants.

What is the bottom line about the cause(s) of ulcerative colitis? The exact cause of UC remains a mystery. It is presently presumed that UC is possibly triggered by some unknown environmental factor(s) in probably genetically predisposed persons who perhaps have a defected (over-reactive) immune system in their colon.

Who Is At Risk For Ulcerative Colitis?

1. Age: Although UC can occur at any age, it is primarily a disease of young people under 30 (often between 15 and 30 years of age), and less frequently in older people. In recent years, the disease has been diagnosed with increasing frequency in children younger than 15 years. The disease in children tends to be more

aggressive than in older kids or young adults, requiring more aggressive treatment plans to get them into remission.

2. Race and ethnicity: Although the disease has initially been reported in white people of European descent particularly of Jewish ancestry, more recently UC has been diagnosed in people of various races and ethnicities.
3. Geographic location: Since the early diagnosed cases of UC occurred in Europe, the disease has been diagnosed in various countries world-wide.
4. Gender: UC appears to affect both men and women. Women with UC may find their symptoms are worse during their menstrual cycle.
5. Genetics. *Will my next child get UC as well? What increases the risk of getting UC in another member of the family?* Some scientists believe that UC is a genetically predisposed disease. About 15-30% of patients have a close relative with a similar illness. No one can indisputably tell the likelihood that someone's second child will also get UC. There are no reliable screening tests for predicting who will get UC at present. Certain genes have been linked to UC susceptibility. However, the presence of these genes in a healthy person does not mean that person will eventually develop the disease. Studies on identical twins revealed that only half of identical twins will develop the disease, even though

they share the same genes as their sibling who has the disease. It is clear that there are other risk factors involved beside genes. In other words, it possible that under the right circumstances, an interaction between a gene and specific trigger sets off this uncontrolled inflammation of the colon. The nature of the trigger is unknown and there could be multiple triggers.

Can Ulcerative Colitis Be Prevented?

You cannot prevent ulcerative colitis because the cause is unknown.

What Are The Symptoms Of Ulcerative Colitis?

1. Classic symptoms of UC include diarrhea mixed with blood and abdominal pain. Unpleasant bouts of diarrhea associated with urgency to use the bathroom are frequent at an onset of a flare up. Straining and the feelings of urgency to have a bowel movement are due to the burning sensation caused by the newly developed open erosions and ulcers in the colon. These raw ulcers stimulate the feelings of incomplete emptying of bowel when it actually completely empty and only drops of waste and gas comes out. These straining

episodes are very uncomfortable and are frequent in acute flare ups.

2. Blood in stool from the erosions and ulcers on lining of the colon is a common symptom. Occasionally, a thin film of mucus is seen covering the stool. UC starts with increased frequency of bowel movements. Blood may not be visible in the first few days of UC.
3. Anemia can result from loss of small amounts of blood over a period of time (chronic). Anemia can also result from an acute heavy rectal bleeding. Anemic patients are pale, get fatigued quickly, and complain of dizziness and shortness of breath.
4. Abdominal pain and cramping are frequent and can be very severe. Temporary ease of pain is obtained once waste and gas are released.
5. Patients often pass gas and may have abdominal bloating. This is caused by the gas-producing bacteria which are normal inhabitants in the guts. They are opportunist and grow at the cost of other micro flora in the guts when health of the guts is impaired.
6. Vomiting is seen occasionally.
7. Weight loss is not a common feature of UC but can be seen in some patients experiencing vomiting and loss of appetite. In other words, UC does not impact the body's ability to digest food and absorb nutrients. These functions take place in the stomach and small

intestine. UC affects the colon (large intestine) which primarily absorbs water only.

8. Dehydration is common in patients with UC primarily due to diarrhea. Water absorption is the function of the colon which is targeted by UC. Therefore, water utilization is impaired in patients with UC especially during a flare up. Signs of dehydration may include: dry mouth, sunken eyes, dark circles under eyes, fatigue, loss of appetite, and urinating less frequently with darker than normal urine.
9. Low grade fever may be noticed especially during flare ups.

Which ulcerative colitis symptoms occur first?

Diarrhea is the first sign seen. In mild cases of UC, patients may have 4 to 6 bowel movements a day with or without visible blood. This number increased dramatically during a flare up to 20 times or more bowel movements a day with visible blood and severe cramps.

What is the course of ulcerative colitis? How long before symptoms calm down?

The course of UC can be very unpredictable. Some people experience relatively mild symptoms and long periods of remission. Others suffer more frequent relapses and ongoing ulcerative colitis symptoms. Ulcerative colitis goes through cycles of remission (calming down of symptoms) and flare ups but the disease never entirely disappears for life.

How painful are symptoms of ulcerative colitis?

Pain from UC vary widely from person to person and may range from mild discomfort to severe and unbearable abdominal pain. This variation depends on the severity of inflammation and the extent of involvement of the colon—whether a small segment or the entire colon is affected. During a flare up with a severe attack, people may have 20 bowel movements or more in a day with heavy rectal bleeding and intolerable abdominal pain. Women with UC may find the pain associated with UC worse during their menstrual cycle.

Is it possible that ulcerative colitis changes its course overtime?

Yes. UC is a progressive disease and being a chronic illness, it has ample opportunities to keep changing its course over a lifetime. In some patients, UC may progress in both severity of inflammation and extent of involvement of colon from a small segment of the colon initially, to a major portion despite treatment. The disease may also become less responsive to certain medications. It may respond favorably to a milder medication initially but then less responsive to it overtime which may necessitate stronger drugs.

What warning signs should I look for?

It is a common sense that when caregivers and patients observe any abnormal sign they should seek medical attention. In addition to the diarrhea with blood and abdominal pain, patients with ulcerative colitis are at risk of other possible medical complications. The following is a list of common alarming signs that necessitate immediate medical attention:

1. High fever
2. Severe abdominal pain
3. Frequent episodes of vomiting
4. Blood in the stool
5. Dehydration
6. Frequent bouts of severe diarrhea
7. Weight loss
8. Fistula development on skin (tunnel-like passage) with pus or waste secretion
9. Feeling sad, angry, or depressed
10. Skin disorders such as skin rash and skin tags
11. Painful or inflamed eyes
12. Swollen and painful joints
13. Anemia characterized by pale or yellow discoloration (jaundice) of skin and eye membranes (conjunctiva).
14. Development of side effects from medication. Familiarize yourself with the specific side effects of various drugs used for treatment of ulcerative colitis. They are discussed under "medication" in the treatment section in this book.

15. Immunosuppression caused by the medications is suspected when a person experiences frequent attacks of colds, or showing signs of dormant infections such as chicken pox, tuberculosis, and yeast infection in mouth or other parts of body.

The disease is very unpredictable and may flare up at any time without any warning signs. It is also unpredictable how long the flare up will last.

What Are The Potential Risks Of Having Ulcerative Colitis?

Patients with UC could have both intestinal damage as well as extra-intestinal health issues with varying degrees of intensity from mild to potentially life-threatening complications. Some of these risks can be managed with medication. Others may require surgery or other medical intervention for correction. Although some of these risks are encountered in only a small number of patients with UC, they undoubtedly need to be routinely monitored and watched for.

A. Intestinal Complications of Ulcerative Colitis:

1. *Intestinal damage. What kind and where is the damage in my gut?* UC causes superficial open sores (erosions and ulcers) on the innermost lining (mucosa) of the

large intestine (colon). However, perforation or a hole through the full thickness of the wall of the colon can also occur in long standing cases of UC. Perforated colon can be fatal due to escape of intestinal waste and bacteria into the abdomen and requires an emergency surgery to be corrected. Massive hemorrhage and excruciating abdominal pain and fever are some of the signs of perforated bowel.

2. *Fistulas.* A fistula is an abnormal connecting tract between two adjacent organs such as between the intestine and the bladder, the vagina, or the skin. Intestinal fistulas allow waste and bacteria to pass from the intestine to the other involved structure and require medical or surgical attention to be repaired. Although fistulas may develop in patients with ulcerative colitis, they are rare and encountered only in the most severe forms of UC. This is because the damage caused by UC is limited to the innermost lining of the gut. This is in contrary to damage caused by Crohn's disease which may involve full thickness of the gut. Therefore, intestinal fistulas are more common in patients with Crohn's disease.
3. *Toxic megacolon. What is toxic megacolon and who might get it?* As the name implies, the colon becomes greatly distended "mega size" with gas and waste. On X-rays the colon appears inflated like a balloon. The condition occurs very rarely but requires immediate surgery

when it develops. It is seen in patients with aggressive ulcerative colitis involving a large portion of the colon. Instead of emptying its toxic waste, the affected colon becomes stagnant, distended and its wall is fatigued and loses its tone. Signs of toxic megacolon are severe abdominal pain and fever. Bacteria and toxins can leak through the dilated and thinned wall of the colon into the blood stream causing a very serious toxicity of the blood (toxemia) resulting in high fever. The inflated colon may also burst and spread infection into the abdomen of affected patients. This condition can be fatal if the diseased colon is not surgically removed right away.

4. *Cancer of the colon and rectum. Is a person with ulcerative colitis at high risk for colon cancer? What increases the risk of colon cancer in UC patients?* Yes, cancer of the colon and rectum (colorectal cancer) is a potential risk in patients with ulcerative colitis unless they opt to the surgical removal of the entire colon. It appears that the more the severe the ulcerative colitis involving most of the colon and the more sustained inflammation of the colon, the higher the risk of developing colon cancer. Patients facing the risk of colon cancer are recommended to regularly visit their doctors to undergo colonoscopy for cancer screening to ensure early detection and treatment.
5. *Intestinal blockage. What are the causes and signs of intestinal blockage?* In patients with ulcerative colitis,

intestinal lumen narrowing and blockage can occur due to scar tissue formation within the intestinal wall in response to massive inflammation and damage in the colon. Scar tissue may also develop in tissues surrounding the intestine (peritoneum) following abdominal surgery such as for UC. In these patients, the scar tissue acts like a robe that tightens the neighboring guts and can lead to narrowing or blockage of their lumen. Typical signs of intestinal blockage are vomiting, severe abdominal pain, and inability to pass gas or a bowel movement. Surgery is required to correct intestinal obstruction.

B. Extra-Intestinal Risks of Ulcerative Colitis:

Although UC primarily affects the intestine, secondary complications outside the intestine can be encountered in some patients as an indirect effect of the disease.

1. *Arthritis. How serious is arthritis?* Arthritis or inflammation of the joints can be seen in some patients with UC. Symptoms may range in severity from mild joint pain, stiffness, and swelling of some joints, to a debilitating arthritis associated with loss of flexibility in affected joints. Lower back joints and knee joints involvement can be crippling when severely affected. Arthritis in these patients may be related to the disease

as an extra-intestinal manifestation or may be related to medication side effects such as prednisone which can cause bone loss and subsequent joint pain.

2. *Skin disorders.* Skin rash, skin tags, and canker sores in the mouth can be seen in some patients with UC.
3. *Eye disorders. Can UC causes blindness?* Some patients with UC may experience inflammation of the eye, and glaucoma, with potential loss of vision if left untreated.
4. *Liver disease. What to look for if my liver becomes affected.* Mild scarring of the bile ducts, gallstones, and fatty liver occur in some patients with UC. Affected patients may appear pale or having yellow discoloration of skin and mucous membranes such as of the eyes and gum. Other signs may include loss of appetite, abdominal pain, and vomiting.
5. *Bone loss. Do I need crutches? Am I more prone to suffering from broken bones?* Osteoporosis, or thinness of bones, can be caused directly by UC or as a side effect of long term use of medications. Steroids, in particular, interfere with utilization of calcium which is essential for bone formation. People with osteoporosis are at a higher risk of bone fractures and may experience joint pain.
6. *Weight loss. Why is this?* The small intestine, where absorption of digested nutrients normally takes place, is not affected in patients with UC. The disease affects the colon and the main and only function of the colon

is the absorption of water. Malnourishment and weight loss are therefore not very common in people with UC. However, they can be seen in patients with long standing and difficult to control forms of UC. In these patients, weight loss is primarily due to loss of appetite because of severe abdominal pain and the unpleasant feelings of frequent visits to the bathroom. Eating just isn't a priority for people in such circumstances. Weight loss may also in part due to frequent diarrhea. Weight loss in these cases is because the digested food is not staying long enough in the small intestine to be fully absorbed. In other words the transit time of food through the digestive tract is too quick for the nutrients to be fully utilized by the body. Vomiting could also be another reason but vomiting is not commonly encountered in patients with UC.

7. *Mental and emotional effects and quality of life. Where can I get emotional support from?* UC can affect more than a person's physical health. It can affect the patient's mental and emotional well-being as well. Quality of life will be impacted and will be reflected on almost every area of one's life from work, academic, family, to social life. Many people with UC struggle with body image. Frequent and urgent bouts of diarrhea are common in flare ups and are often associated with pain. Multiple trips to the bathroom can be exhausting especially at night or early in the morning before going

to work or school. There is also the concern of not finding a bathroom en route or not even making it to the bathroom. Frequent visits to the bathroom while at work can interrupt duties and affect job performance. It can be used by other employees as a reason for discrimination and can lead to a loss of self-worth and confidence. Patients may feel embarrassed, sad, angry, or even depressed. Refer to page 157 in this book for more details on these issues and where to get help.

8. *Dehydration. What are the signs of dehydration?* Dehydration is common in patients with UC due to loss of fluid mainly through diarrhea, not drinking enough, and partly due to vomiting. Signs of dehydration include sunken eyes, dark circles under eyes, reduced urine output, dark urine, and fatigue.
9. *Anemia. Do I need blood transfusion?* Significant amounts of blood can be lost within a short time during flare ups of UC. Blood can also be lost in the stool in tiny almost invisible amounts persistently over time in patients with UC that is not fully under control. In both situations, loss of blood is significant and anemia will result. Anemia will also result from loss of iron in UC patients. Iron is a major component of the red blood cells so loss of blood associated with rectal bleeding means loss of iron as well. Iron is essential to synthetize new red blood cells. In other words, bone marrow cannot produce red blood cells in iron deficient patients.

Anemic patients appear pale and feel fatigued and their productivity at work is impacted. They may also suffer from dizziness and shortness of breath. Critically anemic people will require blood transfusion.

10. *Multiple medications side effects.* Due to ulcerative colitis being a chronic illness with no known cure except surgery, people with UC are likely to be on life-long medications. Consuming various medications for extended periods of time can increase the risk of severe side effects and may induce other medical problems. Please reference the medications section of this book, page 37, for detailed information on the specific side effects of each drug associated with the treatment of UC.

How Is Ulcerative Colitis Diagnosed?

Diarrhea with blood and abdominal pain that are experienced by patients with UC can mimic the symptoms caused by a number of other illnesses such as infections with bacterial organisms like *Clostridium difficile*, food poisoning due to contamination of food with *E. coli,* and *Salmonella* organisms, and stomach flu virus. It is essential to reach a definitive diagnosis of UC to tailor the proper treatment. However, differentiating these illnesses can be very challenging, time consuming, and frustrating, especially at the onset of the disease. Doctors rely on the following steps to tell the difference between the various illnesses that mirror UC and to reach the conclusive diagnosis of UC.

1. Medical History:

A thorough medical history will provide crucial clues during the diagnostic process of ulcerative colitis. A patient with a long-standing history of diarrhea that does not respond to common anti-diarrhea medications, who has intermittent rectal bleeding for some time, and also has another family member with UC can raise the suspicion of UC.

I am embarrassed to tell everyone what I am experiencing. Accompanying a loved one to the doctor's office can be a very rewarding and relieving experience. A caregiver can provide some useful supplemental information that patients may feel embarrassed or ashamed to talk about, such as the frequency of going to the bathroom and of passing gas. Some patients may also feel inhibited or unwilling to admit certain facts, particularly when it comes to emotional or mental issues. Ulcerative colitis affects young people who may be more concerned about self-image and may feel shy or awkward to tell the full story. Doctors rely on the information given by the patient in order to choose the best course of action. It is essential that the patient be open and tells everything about his/her feelings and struggles. Patients need to realize that doctors are used to hearing about all kinds of disease symptoms and that there is absolutely no reason to be embarrassed.

2. Complete Physical Examination:
Your doctor will need to perform a complete body physical examination which has already initiated by the nurse who checks your temperature, pulse, and blood pressure. Your doctor will examine you from head to toe, including listening to your heart and lungs and checking your eyes, ears, and throat. The doctor will feel your abdomen for tenderness and check the rectum for hemorrhoids or tears.

Next, your physician will recommend some preliminary laboratory tests which will probably include blood, stool, and urine tests to form a picture about the general health of the various body systems. Results of these laboratory tests will also offer basic but vital information that help map the pathway of the diagnostic process and aid additional testing needed to differentiate the various disease conditions.

3. Laboratory Diagnostic Tests:
There are several procedures and tests that are often performed in combination to make the diagnosis of ulcerative colitis. Some of the tests are performed to eliminate certain disease conditions with similar symptoms. Other tests are

used to look for evidence of UC. Each procedure and test provides valuable information. The results of these tests are collectively utilized to make a definitive diagnosis. In other words, there is no single test to ensure a clear cut diagnosis of UC. Diagnosing UC is a complex process and that may take several days or weeks to reach the correct diagnosis. The disease can be extremely challenging to diagnose in some patients. Below are common diagnostic tests.

i. Blood tests. Blood tests are performed routinely to check the basic values of several blood elements. Examples include:

a. *Testing for anemia:* Both hemoglobin values and red blood cell counts are examples of routinely performed tests to check for anemia.
b. *To detect systemic inflammation:* Inflammation and infection elevate the white blood cells count. Elevated C-reactive proteins test and erythrocyte sedimentation rate (ESR) or SED rate test provide confirmation of systemic inflammation, the hallmark of inflammatory bowel disease, like ulcerative colitis and Crohn's disease.
c. *To measure values of trace minerals and electrolytes:* Blood tests will be indicated to measure values of various minerals, such as iron in anemic patients, and electrolytes, including sodium and potassium in dehydrated patients, to consider their shortages in the treatment plan.

d. *To monitor function of various organs:* Blood chemistry tests are used to monitor the function of vital organs like the liver, the kidney, and the pancreas.
e. *To detect exposure to other ailments:* Additional blood tests (serology) are performed as necessary to check for exposure to certain diseases such as HIV, the virus that causes AIDS, and hepatitis virus.
f. *To monitor nutritional status:* Protein and blood glucose values are checked and monitored to correct levels.
g. *Blood tests are also performed to test for food allergies.*

ii. Stool tests. Stool tests are routinely performed in patients with diarrhea to identify various causes of diarrhea such as infection with harmful bacteria like *Salmonella, E. coli, Clostridium difficile* or parasites like *Giardia*. Stool tests are also used to monitor the presence of blood in the stool. Patients with ulcerative colitis that are not yet under complete control may lose tiny invisible amounts of blood in the stool. Your physician may give you test kits to conveniently use at home for this purpose. It is a simple test yet very informative. Absence of blood in stool indicates no newly developed ulcers and that the disease is well under control.

iii. Urine tests. Urine tests are also routinely performed to reflect on the health of the urinary system. The physical appearance of urine, including clearness and color, along with checking the specific gravity of urine are very useful in this regard. Urine will routinely be tested for presence of blood, sediments like urinary crystals, and other abnormal contents like sugar and protein. Urine culture is indicated to identify causes of urinary tract infections.

Once the list of suspected diseases is shortened, based on the results of the above laboratory tests, more specific testing may be performed to accurately distinguish between very similar diseases like Crohn's disease and ulcerative colitis.

iv. Tissue Biopsy. This is a routine procedure performed during the colonoscopy and upper gastrointestinal endoscopy procedures (see below) in which tiny pieces of the inflamed area of the digestive tract lining are pinched out and examined under the microscope for abnormalities invisible to the naked eye. This examination reveals the nature of damage or inflammation in the biopsied tissues, therefore aiding in eliminating certain diseases and conditions and providing vital information in the diagnosis of ulcerative colitis. Changes seen in tissues under the microscope may reveal features of various conditions such as the exposure to allergens, presence of precancerous cells, exposure to fungal, bacterial, or viral infections, and chronic inflammation. It may also reveal some features indicative of UC or Crohn's disease. Biopsies may also be utilized to monitor the healing progress and response to treatment.

4. *Endoscopic Diagnostic Procedures:* The combination of intestinal endoscopy and biopsy are the most important procedures in confirming the diagnosis of ulcerative colitis.

The endoscope is used to visualize the lining of the esophagus, stomach, and intestines. Specifically, doctors look for erosions, ulcers, and bleeding sites. The endoscope is a long flexible hose-like narrow tube with a tiny light and video camera on its tip. Images of the digestive tract lining are viewed on a television screen. Laxatives or enemas are usually taken prior to the procedure to clean out the digestive system for clear viewing

a. *Colonoscopy.*

This is currently the gold standard procedure for confirming damages caused by ulcerative colitis. It is also used to monitor response to treatment. The endoscope tube is inserted through the rectum to inspect the entire length of the colon and the very end of the small intestine (terminal ileum) when possible.

A full colonoscopy is usually performed under sedation or short general anesthesia to avoid any discomfort. It is especially necessary in young patients struggling with pain to avoid possible accidental perforation of the colon by the endoscope tube.

b. *Sigmoidoscopy.*

This test is similar to a colonoscopy but the tube is shorter and is therefore used to view the lower portion of the colon (sigmoid colon). The procedure is usually well tolerated and is done as an outpatient procedure without sedation. For safety reasons, only sigmoidoscopy will be performed in patients with a swollen colon that does not allow passing of the scope with ease. Otherwise, a complete colonoscopy is the preferred procedure.

c. *Upper Gastrointestinal Endoscopy.*

Endoscopy procedure can also be used to view the lining of the esophagus, stomach, and beginning of the small intestine. For this purpose, the endoscope in inserted through the mouth and the procedure can be performed under sedation or short general anesthesia.

d. Capsule Endoscopy.

Colonoscopy and endoscopy are good procedures to view the lower and the upper ends of the digestive tract respectively. The middle part of the gut is not fully accessible by either of these procedures. Capsule endoscopy is a modern electronic technique that utilizes a capsule encased a miniature camera the size of a large vitamin capsule. The patient swallows the capsule. As the camera capsule travels through the digestive system a video signal is transmitted to a recording belt and the images are analyzed on a computer monitor until the capsule comes out in the stool approximately 8 hours later. Because the patient has to swallow the capsule, this procedure is not recommended for patients with suspected intestinal stricture, narrowing, or obstruction. It is also not recommended for patients who experience vomiting.

Endoscopy is more useful than X-rays in detecting damages caused by ulcerative colitis on the lining of the rectum because the procedure allows visual observation of the damage. It also allows the biopsy sampling of affected areas. X-rays, however, are non-invasive and are useful for detecting certain abnormalities in the digestive tract that do not require the use of endoscopy, such as intestinal obstruction and perforation.

5. *Imaging Diagnostic Techniques:*

   a. *Radiography (plain X-rays)*

Radiographs of the abdomen are commonly used in patients with ulcerative colitis as the initial procedures to screen for abdominal abnormalities in general. Radiographs are more specifically used in UC patients for intestinal abnormalities, such as small bowel obstruction, intestinal perforation, and toxic megacolon.

b. Contrast X-rays.

Barium is a contrast liquid that is commonly used to coat the inside of the digestive tract and to allow for clear visualization of the lining of the stomach and intestines on X-ray films.

Contrast liquids come in various flavors and are either taken orally to view the lining of the stomach and small intestine or are given as an enema to view the lining of the large intestine and the terminal segment of the small intestine (ileum).

Contrast liquids allow see ulcerations on the lining of the stomach and intestine. They help to diagnose abnormal narrowing and obstruction of the bowel and may detect fistulas (tunnel-like passage that connects the intestine to an adjacent organ).

c. Computed Tomography Scan (CT scan).

This is a non-invasive procedure. It utilizes computer imaging and X-ray scanning to produce a series of cross-sectional "slice-by-slice" detailed pictures of the entire abdomen. Health of the intestine can be determined from the resultant three-dimensional images. CT scan is especially helpful in detecting abscesses, intestinal perforations, fistulas, scarring, and intestinal obstruction which are common especially in patients with Crohn's disease. Abscesses are collections of pus in tissues or a cavity.

d. Ultrasound (US) and Magnetic Resonance Imaging (MRI).

These procedures are performed to view internal organs. They are non-invasive procedures that utilize radio-waves that echo back once they strike the internal organs. The echo waves are seen as images and their appearance help in diagnosing the defect such as an abscess, a hole in the gut, or a mass. Magnetic waves will be distorted by the presence of metals in the body. Examples are metal rods used in fixing fractured bones, unless they are stainless steel. It is advisable to inform your doctor if applicable.

Do I have ulcerative colitis or something else? What other diseases cause diarrhea and bleeding?

Exhibited symptoms by individuals with ulcerative colitis can mimic diarrhea and rectal bleeding due to other causes such as the conditions listed below. The tests and procedures discussed above are utilized by doctors to make a definite diagnosis.

1. *Food Poisoning.* Food poisoning remains to be the number one cause of diarrhea in most people. It is caused by ingestion of food contaminated with microbial

toxin or food contaminated with germs like bacteria, viruses, and parasites.

2. *Hemorrhoids, diverticulitis,* and *colorectal cancers.* These conditions cause rectal bleeding and abdominal pain similar to UC but are relatively easier to recognize because of their distinguished appearance on colonoscopy.
3. *Spastic colitis or irritable bowel syndrome (IBS).* This is a very common gastrointestinal disorder with an unknown cause. Similar to ulcerative colitis, IBS affects the large intestine, causing abdominal cramps, pain, gas, and diarrhea. Unlike UC, this syndrome does not cause inflammation of the intestine and thus bears no relationship to UC except for sharing the symptoms above. One hallmark difference between the two conditions is that blood accompanies the diarrhea in patients with UC but not in people with irritable bowel syndrome. IBS does not cause fever (a sign of inflammation) and can be managed through lifestyle changes such as diet modification and stress reduction techniques. Avoiding certain foods such as gluten or other allergens may prevent IBS. Also IBS symptoms may disappear after a person gets rest such as after a short sleep.
4. *The most common disease that mimics ulcerative colitis is Crohn's disease. It has a very similar pattern of diarrhea, bleeding and abdominal pain.*

What are the differences between ulcerative colitis and Crohn's disease?

Crohn's disease is very closely related to ulcerative colitis. It causes very similar symptoms to those exhibited by patients with UC and very similar damages in their intestine. The cause of Crohn's disease is also unknown and could very well be similar to that of UC. Treatment protocol for the two diseases is very similar and overlaps in many of its aspects. Because of the very close similarities between UC and Crohn's disease, the two disorders are collectively included under the term inflammatory bowel disease (IBD). The two diseases differ in the following features:

1. *Damage level.* The intestinal ulcers in people with Crohn's disease can extend through the full thickness of the intestinal wall rather than superficially on the innermost lining of the intestine as seen in patients with UC.
2. *Sites attacked.* Ulcerative colitis affects the large intestine (colon and rectum) only. This fact differentiates UC from Crohn's disease, which can affect multiple parts of the digestive tract; namely the mouth, stomach, and small and large intestines.

   However, telling UC and Crohn's disease apart is not as easy as it sounds, especially when the ulcerations are confined to the large intestine (colon), a common shared site for both of these diseases. Distinguishing between these two diseases is of upmost importance when it comes to treatment and more specifically, the surgical option.

3. *Fissures or tears around the anus, fistulas (tunnel-like passage), and abscesses.* These damages are common in patients with Crohn's disease and occur rarely, if at all, in patients with ulcerative colitis.
4. *Blood antibody testing.* Special blood tests are also available to help distinguish between UC and Crohn's disease. However, these tests are not one hundred percent reliable. More research is needed to refine these tests and to make them more specific and sensitive.

What Are My Treatment Options?

Ulcerative colitis symptoms can intermittently flare up over the course of a patient's lifetime unless the colon is surgically removed. Patients with mild or moderate attacks of ulcerative colitis can benefit from medical treatment. However, others may contract more aggressive disease that requires surgery.

I. Medical Treatment

Is there a drug that cures ulcerative colitis? Unfortunately, since the cause of UC is still unknown, there is no medication that offers a cure. The ultimate goal of drug therapy in patients with UC is to bring the illness into remission and to keep it there. In other words, medications are used to relieve symptoms of pain and the uncomfortable bouts of diarrhea, to suppress the overactive immune system, and to improve the quality of life for people with UC. There are several medications to achieve these goals which often are used individually or in combination depending on the severity of the illness.

How long will I take these medications? Because there is no cure for the disease, patients with medically manageable UC will likely take these medications for life to remain in remission. Patients should not stop taking these medications on their own even when UC is in remission for long periods. Doctors may modify the treatment plan to a maintenance level to decrease the potential for future flare ups.

Can I take over-the-counter medications? Patients should not take any medications including aspirin, ibuprofen, vitamins, and herbal supplements, without consulting their doctor first. Over the counter medications may potentiate or negatively interact with medications you are currently taking for UC.

What are the benefits and risks of ulcerative colitis drugs? Since UC is an inflammatory condition, medications used to treat UC are primarily anti-inflammatory drugs. In other words, they suppress the body's immune system to stop the inflammation that causes the disease. So, while these drugs have the benefits of putting UC in remission, many of them make patients susceptible to other infections. Taking these medications for long periods of time can increase the risk of their side effects and sometimes can create other health problems as well. Some of the side effects of these drugs are similar to symptoms of UC such as diarrhea and abdominal pain.

Proper monitoring of patients who are taking these medications is critical. This involves regular doctor visits, frequent blood testing, and prompt reporting by patients of worrisome symptoms. It should be emphasized that the benefits of these medications far outweigh the risk of their use and the risk of having active UC.

What are the challenges of long- term medical treatment for ulcerative colitis? Non-compliance or not adhering to the treatment plan as prescribed is a common challenge to patients of all chronic diseases. Taking medications over an extended period of time can be frustrating for some patients. High cost of medications and the inconvenience of taking them on a schedule constitute additional challenges. Once in remission, patients generally tend to avoid taking medications. Experiencing the unpleasant side effects such as weight gain, mood swings, and acne associated with use of corticosteroids are other deterring causes. Young people and people with psychiatric problem are less likely to adhere to the medical schedule and are hard to convince about the importance of taking medications.

When may it be time to switch medications? Ulcerative colitis is a lifelong illness. Medications that are used to treat or maintain UC in remission are in a constant state of change. New medications are being introduced and tested all the time. Switching from one medication to another may become necessary during the course of treatment for various reasons, including:

1. Poor response to the initially selected medication.
2. The appearance of worrisome side effects associated with use of that medication.
3. In some patients, a particular drug may stop working. UC may change dramatically over time in both severity of inflammation and extent of involvement of colon and may become less responsive to certain medications. In other words, UC may initially respond favorably to a particular medication but becomes less responsive to it over time and necessitates stronger drugs.
4. Some medications are meant to be for short-term use such as corticosteroids. They are used to attain a status of remission and patients are then switched to different maintenance medications.
5. Once remission is achieved, doctors may taper certain medications or switch medication to safer types to decrease the potential of drug side effects.
6. Marketing new drugs that are more efficacious in controlling the disease with lesser side effects.

Can I stop taking the medications once a state of remission is maintained? No. Ulcerative colitis goes in cycles of remission and flare ups, but never really disappears. Therefore, it is very important for patients with UC to continue taking medications as prescribed by their doctor even if the disease is inactive. Stopping medication can cause the UC to flare up.

What medications are used to treat ulcerative colitis? There are several medications to control symptoms of UC that are often used in a combination depending on the severity of illness. Medications for treatment of UC fall under one of three major groups of drugs: anti-inflammatories (aminosalicylates and corticosteroids), immunomodulators, and biologic therapies. There are other miscellaneous medications, but they are used as a complementary rather than replacement to the major groups of medications.

Ulcerative Colitis Medications: Benefits, Risks, and Side Effects

1. Anti-Inflammatory Medications:

As the name implies, anti-inflammatory drugs help to stop the inflammation. They include the aminosalicylates and corticosteroids.

A. *Aminosalicylates: the first line therapies of ulcerative colitis*

Drugs in this group are commonly used as a first line of therapy in patients with relatively mild to moderate symptoms of UC, and for maintaining remission. They are also used in combination with other drugs to treat moderate and severe attacks of UC.

Commonly used aminosalicylates:

Commonly used drugs in this group are sulfasalazine (Azulfidine), olsalazine (Dipentum), balsalazide (Colazal, Lialda) and mesalamine (Asacol, Pentasa, Apriso, Canasa, Rowasa).

How are aminosalicylates supplied?

These medications can be given by mouth in the forms of tablet or liquid. Patients who have UC limited to the lower part of the colon or in the rectum may take these medications in suppository form or as an enema.

Every patient with ulcerative colitis will have a taste of the aminosalicylates:

These drugs have the least amount of side effects in comparison to other medications used in treatment of UC, and are therefore considered the safest of drugs for this purpose.

Side effects of the safest medications for ulcerative colitis:
Each drug in this group carries its own list of side effects but, in general, medications in this group may cause nausea, abdominal pain, headache, anemia, dizziness, skin rashes, sore throat, flu-like symptoms, and diarrhea.

Sulfasalazine (Azulfidine) may turn urine a bright orange-yellow. In males, sulfasalazine can cause a temporary low sperm count. Some of these medications can also make a person more sensitive to the sun. Some reports on these medications describe side effects on the kidneys and pancreas.

Not all ulcerative colitis flare ups would respond well to treatment with aminosalicylates. They rather necessitate more potent anti-inflammatory drugs to become under control. For such patients, the second line of treatment would be the corticosteroids.

B. Corticosteroids the fast acting drugs to stabilize flare ups

Corticosteroids are the next level of anti-inflammatory drugs used in treating ulcerative colitis and are often indicated when symptoms of UC are more severe. Steroids are fast-acting and potent anti-inflammatory medications, making them extremely valuable, especially at the onset of the disease and during periodic symptom flare-ups to calm the attacks quickly.

Corticosteroids are meant to be for short term use:
Corticosteroids are not appropriate for long-term maintenance therapy because of their serious side effects. Once symptoms of ulcerative colitis are under control, the aminosalicylates listed above are often used to keep patients in remission and the corticosteroids are gradually tapered off.

Commonly used corticosteroids:
Prednisone (Deltasone), methylprednisolone (Medrol), hydrocortisone, and budesonide (Entocort EC) are examples of commonly used medications in this group.

These medications are tailored to all kinds of ulcerative colitis:
Corticosteroids are manufactured in different forms. Some corticosteroids can be taken as tablets by mouth, others as liquid given by intravenous injection, such as in severe cases of UC. Other forms of steroids can be administered as an enema, suppository, or foam delivered to the rectum. Rectal steroids are particularly useful when UC involves the lower part of the large intestine, and have fewer side effects than oral or injectable corticosteroids.

Budesonide capsules are corticosteroids designed to work only in the intestine, thus reducing the potential for systemic side effects.

Corticosteroids will make you eat more and drink more among other side effects:

Side effects of steroids include water retention in body tissues. Patients using steroids appear to have a puffy, round face commonly known as "moon face" or "facial mooning" due to water retention in the face. Prednisone intake causes increased appetite and consequent weight gain. Other side effects of steroids are nausea and vomiting, stomach irritation, headaches, night sweats, dizziness, and mood and personality changes (mood swings).

Long term use of prednisone impairs the utilization of calcium by bones. Calcium is necessary for bone growth and strength. Consequently, joint pain, bone thinning (osteoporosis), and fractures of bones can occur in patients with long-term use of steroids. In children, long-term use of steroids can impair or block their bone growth, and children appear short or stunted in their height.

Prolonged use of steroids may also cause acne, stretch marks on skin, increased facial and body hair, diabetes, cataracts, glaucoma, and high blood pressure. However, the most concerning side effect of long term use of steroids is suppression of the immune system, with increased susceptibility to infection with germs such as bacteria and viruses.

Children and growing young adult patients need to be closely monitored by their physician while on steroids.

Our body naturally produces a corticosteroid-like hormone called cortisol. The production of cortisol will be suppressed or stop in patients taking steroids medications. Therefore, one should not stop taking steroid medications abruptly. Following its initial use, the dose of steroids needs to be tapered off gradually and carefully according to recommendations by your physician so that the body has time to ramp up its natural cortisol production.

Some ulcerative colitis patients flare up once they stop taking the steroids. This means they have become dependent on steroids. Corticosteroids are not meant to be for long term use due to extreme side effects so immunomodulators would be the next therapy to treat these patients.

2. Immunomodulators:

Who benefits from immunomodulators?
Immunomodulators are used in patients who are not able to wean themselves off corticosteroids or are no longer responding to steroids. These are usually patients with severe and persistent UC. The immunomodulator drugs are used to modulate or "calm-down" the immune system. They are potent medications and could impair the function of the immune system. To give you an idea of their potency, drugs like cyclosporine are used in patients with organ transplants to prevent rejection of implanted organ. Some of the immunomodulators

drugs are slow acting and may take weeks to produce an effect. Therefore, they are often used in combination with corticosteroids to quickly control the flare up symptoms and attain remission.

Examples of immunomodulator drugs:
Azathioprine (Imuran, Azasan), 6-mercaptomurine (6-MP, Purinethol), Cyclosporine A (Sandimmune, Neoral), and tacrolimus (Prograf) are some of the commonly used immunomodulators.

How are immunomodulators supplied?
Some immunomodulators are prepared for oral use and others are given by injection.

Beware of the serious side effects of immunomodulators:
These drugs are not for every patient with ulcerative colitis:
Immunomodulators can cause serious side effects such as bone marrow suppression, kidney and liver damage, and lymphoma (cancer of the lymph nodes). These drugs can induce generalized and extensive immune suppression thus lessening the body's ability to combat infection and consequently lead to an increased risk of infection with bacteria, fungi and viruses. Other side effects include nausea, vomiting, diarrhea,

loss of appetite, increased hair growth on face and body, acne, headaches, tremors and tingling in fingers and toes, possible seizures, restlessness, thickening of gums, unusual bleeding or bruising, flu-like symptoms, and sore throat. High blood pressure is another risk and needs to be monitored regularly when taking these drugs.

Frequent blood testing is required to check the levels of these drugs in the body and to monitor their possible toxic effects on the various organs as well.

Patients taking corticosteroids or immunomodulators should discuss with their doctors beforehand any required vaccinations for the entry of school or when traveling to other countries, since the immune system is being altered by the medications consumed. The family doctor will be the best person to advise you whether to have the required vaccines or that certain precautions needed to be taken first.

Patients with UC who fail to respond to the above traditional therapies become good candidates for biologic therapies.

3. Biologic Therapies:

Biologic therapies, or biologic response modifiers, are drugs that target enzymes, proteins, and cells that play a key role in inflammation and inhibit their action. Consequently they calm down the inflammatory response. These medications will not cure ulcerative colitis but help reduce the inflammation and induce a status of remission. Biologic therapies are the newest class of drugs used for patients with UC. These drugs often become less effective over time.

Examples of biologic therapy drugs:
Adalimumab (Humira), certolizumab pegol (cimzia), natalizumab (Tysabri) and infliximab (Remicade) are examples of drugs in this group.

How are biologic therapies supplied?
Various forms of these drugs can be given orally, intravenously, via suppository, or through an enema.

The miracles and risks of biologic therapies: Are they suitable for every ulcerative colitis patient?
Unlike immunomodulators, biologic therapies do not suppress the entire body's immune system. Instead they target certain elements of the immune system. They are potent drugs to achieve remission from UC, but can have some serious risks associated with their use like fatal infections. People taking these drugs can easily contract infection by contact with people who are ill such as with upper respiratory tract

infection. They also cause increased susceptibility to infection with dormant germs that cause tuberculosis (TB), fungal infections, and sepsis, a very dangerous infection of the blood. Using Remicade may increase risk of developing lymphoma (cancer of lymph nodes), breast and colon cancer, skin cancer, and autoimmune disorders (such as a lupus-like syndrome). Other side effects are fever, coughing, sweating, and shortness of breath. Because of their side effects, these drugs are spared for patients who fail to respond to or cannot tolerate the more conventional medications.

The side effects of these drugs need to be weighed against their benefits in attaining remission. These drugs are given under a strict health monitoring program. Your doctor will fully evaluate your health status prior to placing you on these drugs. Special tests such as the tuberculin test need to be performed prior to the use of these medications to clear the recipient of dormant TB infection.

Entyvio (vedolizumab), a monoclonal antibody type of drug, was recently approved to treat ulcerative colitis and Crohn's disease. It is given by injection to prohibit the migration of inflammatory cells across blood vessels into inflamed areas of the intestine. The most common side effects in patients treated with Entyvio include headache, joint pain, nausea, and fever. The most serious risks associated with Entyvio include more serious infections, hypersensitivity, infusion-related reactions, and hepatotoxicity (damage to liver cells). Health care professionals should monitor patients on Entyvio for any new onset or worsening of neurological signs and symptoms.

4. Complementary and Alternative Therapies for Ulcerative Colitis:

Complimentary therapies include antibiotic medication, dietary modifications, and stress management. They are used in addition to the traditional medications for treatment of UC rather than as replacements.

A. *Antibiotics. Do they cure ulcerative colitis?*

No bacterial organism has been identified to cause UC. However, bacteria tend to overgrow in the intestine when health of the intestine is compromised, as in people with active UC. Some bacteria cause gas production and strong smell in stool.

The most commonly used antibiotic for this purpose is metronidazole (Flagyl). In addition to its use in acute flare ups, Flagyl is commonly used as a maintenance medication for oral use in some UC patients. Flagyl may cause nausea, vomiting, abdominal discomfort, a metallic taste in the mouth, headaches, tingling in the hands and feet, and may also darken the urine.

The other commonly used antibiotic is ciprofloxacin (Cipro). Cipro is safer than Flagyl and its side effects are rare. Cipro side effects include nausea, vomiting, restlessness, and abdominal pain.

These antibiotics are usually used at the onset of UC to fight bacteria that can cause secondary complications such as abscess formation. These antibiotics may also help control inflammation by reducing bacteria in the intestine and suppressing the immune system.

B. ***Dietary Management.***

I have no appetite to eat, or I throw up every time I eat. What are the alternatives?

Loss of appetite is common in patients with UC especially during a flare up. For very bad attacks of ulcerative colitis, dietary therapy may include consumption of elemental formula directly by mouth or through a feeding tube. The oral dietary formulas consist of predigested nutrients that will be completely absorbed by the intestine without waste production. These dietary formulas will give the patient's large intestine a rest. Other formulas can be given by intravenous catheters or central lines and are especially useful in patients who have no appetite as well those that are vomiting.

What should I eat or avoid eating while having a flare up of ulcerative colitis? What dietary changes and lifestyle strategies should I make to ease symptoms?

Beware of foods that worsen symptoms. Simple dietary changes can prove to be very useful in easing the diarrhea and the abdominal pain. No specific foods or nutrients have been found to cause UC, keep it in remission, or cure it. Many patients share a particular food that worsens symptoms of UC particularly when experiencing a flare up. However, it is never the same food for all patients. Therefore, there is no one recommended diet for all UC patients. Some of the problematic foods that provoke the unpleasant symptoms include dairy products, spicy food, caffeine, alcohol, carbonated drinks, sugars, red meat, and high fiber foods like beans, popcorn, bran, seeds, nuts, fresh fruits and vegetables like cabbage, and cauliflower. High-fat food, fried, and greasy food including rich cream sauces, butter, and many fast food choices may also worsen symptoms. Also, eating small meals more frequently rather than large meals two or three times a day can make a difference.

Foods that make symptoms better:

Foods that seem to be well tolerated by ulcerative colitis patients may include food with soluble fibers such as oatmeal, rice, applesauce, bananas, fish, and yogurt.

Personalizing your meal recipe to avoid triggers:
It is common sense to stay away from food that bothers you or aggravates symptoms of your colitis. You can create your own list of triggering diets by keeping a daily diary of what was eaten and intensity of symptoms and pain level you experienced that day.

Get help with a dietary recipe:
Work with your dietician or doctor to review your list of consumed food and your symptoms. A dietitian can help you create recipes based on your specific needs and make sure that you are getting enough nutrients with a variety of healthy foods. The Crohn's & Colitis Foundation of America Web site lists a number of recipes that may suit your situation (www.ccfa.org)

C. Fluids.

What kind of fluids is best to drink?
Patients with ulcerative colitis lose a considerable amount of fluid and essential electrolytes through diarrhea and consequently may become dehydrated and weak. During warmer seasons or when engaging in physical activity, more fluid and trace elements loss occur through sweating. Drinking plenty of fluids before and after your workout is essential to prevent dehydration.

Adequate fluid intake is vital to the health of patients with ulcerative colitis, especially young children. Dehydration can adversely affect the kidneys. Signs of dehydration are dry mouth, dark lines below eyes, and reduced urine output. Also, dehydrated patients feel weak and tired.

Keeping track of what you drink and monitoring experienced level of pain and frequency of diarrhea is of utmost importance in this regard. Avoid drinking too hot or too cold beverages. Have drinks with essential electrolytes supplement to compensate for trace elements lost in diarrhea, sweating, and exercise especially in hot weather. Eating table salt in the diet or salt tablets encourages drinking more fluids and retention of water in body. It is a good practice to drink fluids throughout the day instead of drinking large amounts once or twice a day. Have a bottle of water with you at all times whether you're at work, in school, at home, or on the playground. Make it a habit to have a sip of water every time you see the bottle.

D. Supplement Intake.

Do I need to be concerned about nutritional deficiencies because of my ulcerative colitis?

Always follow your doctor's recommendations and do not take any medication or supplement on your own without first consulting your dietitian and doctor.

i. Multivitamins, minerals, antioxidants, omega fatty acids, and probiotics can be helpful and energizing. These supplements are not substitutes for UC medications. They are necessary to compensate for loss in diarrhea, especially in children and young adults whose long-term growth and development requires substantial nutrition.

ii. Iron is essential to help the body produce red blood cells. Low iron levels are encountered in patients who have lost considerable amounts of blood due to rectal bleeding. Affected patients are commonly anemic. Several iron products are on the market for fast or slow release of iron. Commonly supplied forms of iron are liquids for daily oral use or by intravenous injection in patients with critically low iron levels. Prenatal multivitamin tablets are rich in iron and can be used for this purpose. Side effects of iron supplements include nausea, vomiting, staining of teeth, darkened urine, stomach pain and heartburn, constipation, and dark tarry stools. Stomach irritation and nausea can be alleviated by taking slow release iron tablets instead of regular iron forms. Taking iron with meals also helps reduce its irritating effect on the stomach.

iii. Vitamin D and calcium are essential elements for overall good health and bone and muscle health in particular. Bone thinning (osteoporosis) is a common complication in patients with ulcerative colitis. Impaired utilization of calcium can also occur as a side effect of long term use of corticosteroids in treatment of UC. Vitamin D is needed to absorb calcium in the intestine. Daily supplements of vitamin D and calcium may be needed by some patients with UC to prevent osteoporosis. Other bone boosting strategies are exercise, consumption of calcium and vitamin D rich diets, bone strengthening medications like risedronate and alendronate, and limiting bone weakening medications like steroids. Regular testing of bone density by your doctor and measuring levels of vitamin D and calcium in the blood are good for this purpose. Consult with your doctor if you are facing a risk of osteoporosis.

iv. Bacteria of different kinds are normally present in the gut of a healthy person in certain proportions. Bacterial populations are often altered in the inflamed gut of patients with UC. In these patients, bad bacteria that cause gas and inflammation in the gut overgrow the good bacteria that aid in digestion. Probiotics contain the good bacteria and are needed to regulate or balance the bacterial micro flora in the intestines. Various probiotics products are available. These healthy bacteria are commonly found in yogurt yet in smaller numbers. Probiotics products may be taken by mouth in various forms such as liquid or capsules.

E. Management of stress.

How to manage my stress, loneliness, and sad feelings?
Although stress does not cause ulcerative colitis, stress management may help healing, ease symptoms of ulcerative colitis, and improve quality of life. Living with a chronic illness such as UC can cause an individual to become depressed, anxious, and socially isolated. Untreated depression and anxiety can certainly make life less enjoyable, restrict or interfere with one's daily activities, and can worsen symptoms of UC.

People with ulcerative colitis may experiment with various relaxing techniques that best work for them to reduce the effects of stress. These may include light exercise, deep breathing, yoga, meditation, tai chi, hypnosis, swimming, walking, massage, listening to soft relaxing music, warm baths, or any other activity that you enjoy. Having a positive attitude and letting things go help a lot. You can do these exercises at home without having to worry about being near a bathroom. Invite a friend to watch a movie together or read an interesting book.

To avoid suffering in isolation one can get involved in group activities such as summer camps for kids with UC run by the Crohn's & Colitis Foundation of America, participate in fundraising efforts for research on UC, and other mood boosting activities. Volunteer some of your time working for a church, a hospital, a charity organization, an animal shelter, or a homeless shelter. Helping others will have the added bonus of helping you.

Am I getting the support I deserve? Where can I get emotional support from? Can I get one-on-one support?

Ulcerative colitis is a chronic disease that can cause anxiety and emotional distress in addition to affecting physical health. Emotional support is crucial for patients with UC. It also helps to keep the illness symptoms under control. Treat yourself well.

Emotional support can be obtained from a number of sources that include doctors and other mental health professionals, friends, family, loved ones, religious leaders, teachers, school counselor, and Crohn's and Colitis support advocate groups. The bottom line is to vent your feelings and make your spouse, friends, and relatives aware of your suffering. They may not be able to fix your problems but it will be helpful for them to understand your emotions while struggling with UC. Simply saying that you don't feel like yourself can help you feel better. Joining a support group can be a great way to learn more about UC and also meet people who have been through similar experiences. They may have good suggestions or experiences that perfectly fit your situation. Moreover, you will certainly find reassurance in just knowing that there are other people who feel the same way you do. One can physically attend local meetings or chat online with patients who are going through the same illness and share and receive feedback on their concerns. The Crohn's & Colitis Foundation of America website is a great place to start. Everyone needs support at some point. Do not feel ashamed or afraid to ask for help. You are not the only one with this illness. Thousands of people are experiencing what you are going through. UC cannot be medically cured but stress and depression can.

F. Blood Transfusion.

When is blood transfusion needed? What are the involved benefits and risks?

This procedure involves transmitting blood from a donor and given through an intravenous infusion to a person who needs it. Patients with UC can lose considerable amounts of blood especially during a flare up and as a result, may become anemic. They may also lose invisible tiny amounts of blood in stool, but continuously over time, when their UC is not fully under control. Even though there is strict screening and testing of donated blood for various infectious diseases such as HIV (the virus that causes AIDS) and hepatitis virus, there is still a slim risk of infection with these viruses following blood transfusion. In urgent cases where cross matching is not done, reactions can occur when donor blood type is not compatible. Fever and chills can also occur as side effects from blood transfusion.

G. Alternative Therapies.

Are there alternative therapies for ulcerative colitis?

Therapies other than traditional medications, which include acupuncture, Chinese herbs, hypnosis, homeopathic remedies, Ginseng, and Aloe Vera, have been attempted and studied but on a limited basis. Although some of these therapies seem to help some patients, there is not enough data at present to make a sound recommendation for their use in the treatment of UC. Because of the limited experience in using herbs in western medicine, some doctors are hesitant about recommending herbal supplements to patients. Other doctors are skeptical about the positive effects of herbs or even fearful about unknown side effects and their possible interactions with conventional UC medications. Some of the alternative therapies can be expensive and may not be covered by health insurance plans.

H. Contraceptives.

Can oral contraceptive help my pain?

Women with ulcerative colitis may find their symptoms are worse during their menstrual cycle. Oral contraceptive and PMS medications may provide some relief but talking to your doctor before taking any of these medications or any other over the counter medications like aspirin and ibuprofen is highly recommended.

I. Fecal Microbial Transplantation

This involves infusion via enemas of human stool (bowel movement) from a healthy donor to a patient with UC. The idea is to restore the normal micro flora in guts of UC patients. While a few doctors advocated this approach as promising in achieving remission, many are hesitant to recommend it.

II. Surgical Treatment Of Ulcerative Colitis

Medications are usually the first step in treating patients with UC. When a medical approach is not successful for controlling UC, the surgical treatment becomes a viable option to consider.

Ulcerative colitis surgeries: Benefits and risks

Surgery can be a cure for patients with UC. Unlike Crohn's disease which can affect any part of the digestive tract from mouth to anus and which can resurface after surgery in new areas in the remaining parts of the digestive system, UC affects the colon and rectum only. Therefore UC can generally be "cured" by surgical removal of the colon and rectum because there is no remaining tissue for ulcerative colitis to attack. Patients return to normal life and activity with a superior quality of life.

Do I need surgery for my UC?

The following patients are considered ideal candidates for surgical removal of the colon:

1. Patients whose traditional medications including biologic therapies fail to bring UC into remission.
2. Patients with heavy rectal bleeding.
3. Patients with perforated or ruptured colon.
4. Patients with severely distended colon with gas, waste, and bacteria (toxic megacolon).
5. Patients with severe disabling colitis.
6. Patients with possible risk of cancer. Colon cancer is a potential risk in patients with ulcerative colitis, especially in people with repeated relapses over time and in patients where most of the colon is extensively damaged. These patients may need to consider the risk of colon cancer in deciding the medical versus surgical options of treatment.
7. Patients already having precancerous signs or cancerous changes in the colon.

What should I consider before committing myself to surgery for my colitis?

People faced with the surgical decision should gather as much information as possible about all aspects of the procedure. What does the surgery involve? Is surgery for me? Am I a perfect candidate for surgery? What should I expect after surgery? Here are some people who can help you make that decision:

1. In addition to your doctor, talk to several doctors and nurses who work with colon surgery patients, other colon surgery patients, support groups, and other information resources such as the Crohn's & Colitis Foundation of America.
2. Your life-partner's opinions need to be considered at this time to maintain an intimate relationship, especially if an external pouch needs to be used.
3. Emotional support may become necessary for teenagers wearing bags due to embarrassment, aesthetic reasons, concerns about body image, or declined self-esteem. Appearance is very important for everyone but especially for children and teenagers struggling with ulcerative colitis. For adults, additional post-surgical challenges need to be considered such as intimate relationships, incontinence, social life, and work performance issues. All these issues can seriously impact your life if you allow them to.
4. One has to think seriously that once the colon is surgically removed it is gone forever. One may consider trying the new biological drugs such as Remicade, at least on a temporary basis, and hope for the introduction of more safe targeted therapies in the future.

What does the surgical procedure for ulcerative colitis involve?

The standard surgical procedure for patients with UC involves the removal of the entire large intestine including the colon, rectum, and appendix as well as lining of the anus (Figure 1). The remaining small intestine is then either connected to the anus directly in a one-step surgery or may be temporarily connected to an opening in the groin area (Ileostomy) and then connected to the anus in a later surgery. The choice of these two surgeries depends on health of the anal lining. If the lining is healthy a one-step procedure may be performed. Otherwise, if the lining is extensively inflamed or is showing fissures (small cracks) in it, the two or more step procedure may be elected to give the fissures a chance to heal.

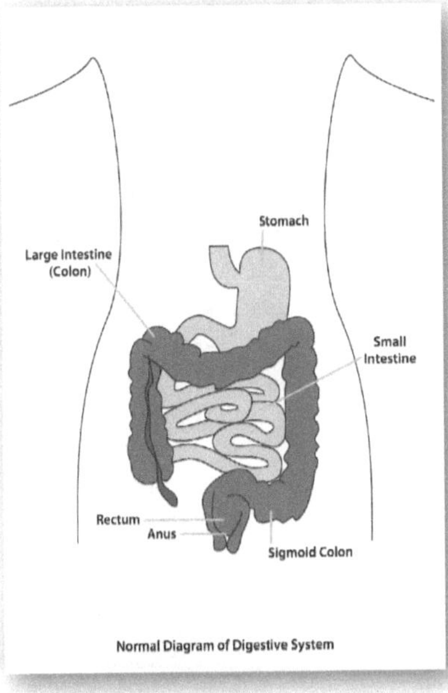

Figure 1. Normal Diagram of Digestive System

1. The one-step surgical procedure (ileo-anal pouch or j-pouch) involves the removal of the entire large intestine at its junction with the small intestine. A pouch is created using the patient's own small intestine. A loop of the last five inches of the small intestine (ileum) is modified surgically to form a sac or pouch located inside the pelvis to replace the rectum and is sewn to the anus. Waste is stored in the pouch and eliminated through the anus in the usual manner. This operational procedure is also called Ileo-anal pouch or j-pouch surgery (Figure 2).

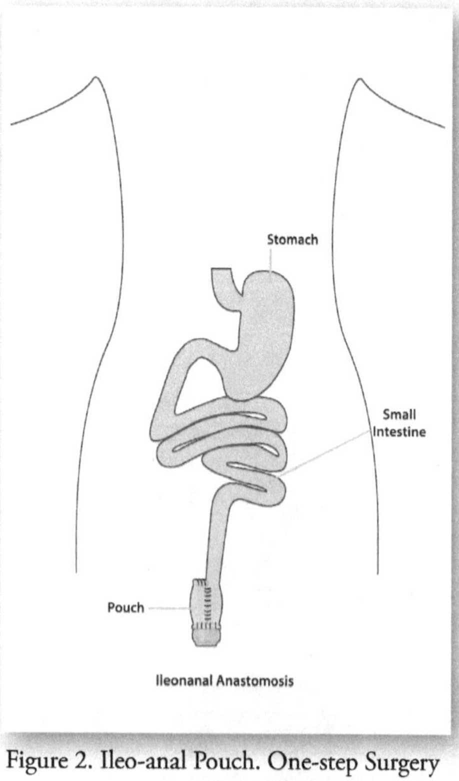

Figure 2. Ileo-anal Pouch. One-step Surgery

2. In the two-step surgical procedure (ileostomy), a small opening about the size of a quarter is constructed above the groin in the lower right wall of the abdomen. This procedure is called temporary ileostomy. Following removal of the large intestine, the small intestine is then connected to this opening. Intestinal waste and gas passes out of this opening and is collected in an external bag (called an ileostomy bag) that is connected to the abdominal hole. There is no odor and the bag fits under clothes easily without being noticed by others. The patient empties the bag as frequently as necessary. Once inflammation in the lining of the anus is healed a second surgery is performed to attach the end of the pouch to the anal opening and the abdominal opening in the groin area is closed off. Defecation then occurs in the traditional way through the anus.

   In the more popular two step surgery, an internal pouch is used instead of the external disposable bag. In this procedure, the last part of the small intestine can be surgically modified to form a pouch or reservoir (Koch pouch) that stays within the abdomen and is connected to the hole in the groin as mentioned above (Figure 3). A nipple valve is constructed around the opening in the groin which allows the patient to empty the pouch by inserting a tube through the abdominal opening to drain the waste. A small bandage is used to cover the valve. Once the anal lining is healed a second surgery is performed to attach the pouch to the anal opening and the abdominal opening in the groin area is closed off. Defecation then occurs in the traditional way through the anus.

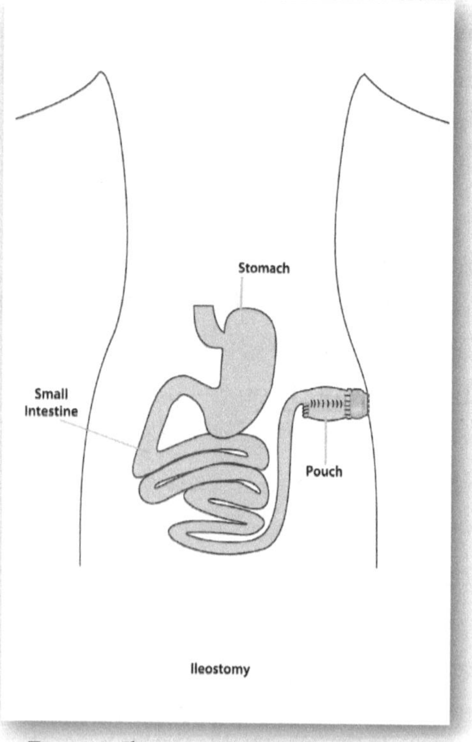

Figure 3. Ileostomy. Two-step Surgery

Post-surgical complications and challenges:

There are possible complications following surgery for ulcerative colitis.

1. *Pouchitis.* The most common post-surgical complication in UC patients is inflammation of the pouch called pouchitis. Symptoms of pouchitis include abdominal pain, diarrhea, rectal bleeding, and fever. Patients may reduce the incidence and intensity of pouchitis by irrigating the pouch with saline solutions and taking antibiotics when needed. Frequent inspection of the pouch by your doctor is necessary to detect tissue changes early. Probiotic intake may also help reduce the incidence of pouchitis.
2. *Soft stool.* Bowel movements become more frequent and of liquid consistency than prior to surgery. This is because water is absorbed primarily by the colon. Stool will remain soft for life after surgery but it gradually gets less watery as the small intestine begins to presume the job of absorbing the water.
3. *Fecal leakage.* Due to the liquid nature of waste and the imperfect tone of the anal sphincter right after surgery, leakage of waste through the anus is common and may cause an embarrassing smell and wetness of clothes or skin rash at the buttocks.

4. *Valve problems.* Inability to insert a catheter through the nipple valve (two-step surgery) in some cases will require a second operation to repair the nipple. Occasional leakage of stool around the nipple may also occur.
5. *Other complications* common to abdominal surgeries, in general can include bleeding, infection, delayed healing, scar formation on skin at the surgical site, and adhesions between abdominal tissues leading to stricture or obstruction of the bowel. Other complications may also occur in relation to the anesthesia.

Disclaimer

THE INFORMATION PRESENTED IN THIS overview of ulcerative colitis is presented for educational purpose ONLY. It does not cover all aspects of the disease and is not intended as medical guide, advice, or a substitute to seeking professional medical care. Always consult with your doctor if you have any questions or concerns about your health condition and before taking any medication. The author disclaims any liability for the decisions you make based on this information.

References

The Crohn's & Colitis Foundation of America –web site www.ccfa.org

Everydayhealth.com

Danese, S. & Fiocci, C. (2011). Ulcerative colitis. The New England Journal of Medicine 365:1713-1725.

Hanauer, Stephen B.; William Sandborn (2001). Management of Crohn's disease in adults. American Journal of Gastroenterology **96** (3): 635–643.

Gut Feelings

Langan RC, Gotsch PB, Krafczyk MA, Skillinge DD (November 2007).Ulcerative colitis: diagnosis and treatment. American family physician**76** (9): 1323–1330.

Geerling BJ, Dagnelie PC, Badart-Smook A, Russel MG, Stockbrügger RW, Brummer RJ (2000). Diet as a risk factor for the development of ulcerative colitis. The American journal of gastroenterology **95** (4): 1008–1013.

Fedorak Richard (2010). Probiotics in the Management of ulcerative colitis. Gastroenterology & Hepatology **6** (11).

Silverman MS, Davis I, Pillai DR (2010). Success of self-administered home fecal transplantation for chronic Clostridium difficile infection. Clin. Gastroenterol. Hepatol. **8** (5): 471–3.

Greenstein AJ, Janowitz HD, Sachar DB (1976). The extra-intestinal complications of Crohn's disease and ulcerative colitis: a study of 700 patients. Medicine **55** (5): 401–412.

Podolsky DK (2002). Inflammatory bowel disease. N. Engl. J. Med. **347**(6): 417–29.

Sonnenberg A, McCarty DJ, Jacobsen SJ (1991). Geographic variation of inflammatory bowel disease within the United States. Gastroenterology **100** (1): 143–9.

Doherty GA, Cheifetz AS (2009). Management of acute severe ulcerative colitis. Expert Review of Gastroenterology and Hepatology. 3(4):395–405.

Part II

CHAPTER 2

Gut Feelings

Sam's Early Life:

What was Sam's early life like before contracting ulcerative colitis? Were there any predisposing factors to his illness?

Sam was born on February 7, 1994. He was a handsome boy with dark red hair, bluish- green eyes, and extraordinary long eyelashes. He had a round, white face with prominently blushed cheeks sprinkled with brown freckles. At birth, he weighed 8 pounds and 7 ounces and was 21 inches in length. He was born perfectly healthy by normal vaginal delivery with no complications. People we met in shopping malls always smiled when they saw his beaming face. We received numerous compliments regarding how charming he was. One woman we met in the grocery store said, "Your baby is so gorgeous." When she discovered Sam was a boy, she commented, "Well, he should be a girl because he is so beautiful!"

He was the first child in the family, so he received great amounts of love and attention from us. His mom decided to be a stay-at-home mom in order to raise Sam with her full attention. His dad was a veterinarian. We traveled frequently for vacations. Sam was very much attached to me. He loved to ride in my old truck when I came home from work.

Sam was very playful, energetic, and outgoing all the time. He was always very happy and never bashful. He was recognized as a very intelligent boy from an early age. He always observed and analyzed all that he saw and asked very clever questions. We adored him dearly as any parents would.

He was always heavily involved in activities and hobbies. He took sewing lessons and learned how to make his own pair of pajamas when he was six years. He also learned to play the guitar, which he picked up astonishingly quick. He then expressed interest in playing the harmonica and ended up playing the trumpet in his school and high school bands. He was a little guy with extensive hobbies. At the age of 5, he wanted to take karate. He was first checked out by the instructor to see if karate was a good fit for him at this young age. His mom and I were watching and giggling from the sidelines. The instructor talked to him in a command officer tone. She ordered him to stand tall with his hands at his waist. He replied "Yes." Then, the instructor raised her voice and commanded Sam to say "Yes, Ma'am!" Sam yelped,

"Yes, Ma'am!" and immediately started crying. We burst out laughing. The trainer apologized and suggested to come back in six months when he is more mature. He never let his illness derail his interest in karate and other sports. Six months later, he was enrolled in karate and was rewarded several belts. He also participated in swimming, bicycling, computer games, and racing on his scooter.

He sang all kind of songs including country music and soft rock. I wondered when and where did he hear and learn these songs, because he was still very young. He was very adventurous, brave, and a risk-taker to try anything and everything. In addition to all of this, he had a great sense of humor and a calm and pleasant personality. His illness and frequent hospitalizations interrupted his life and school attendance tremendously, but never deterred from his interests and ambitions in life.

He received his regular doctor visits for health check up on schedule and had most, but not all, of his immunization shots on time. This is because he contracted his serious illness at an early age and he was placed on immunosuppressive medications. For this reason, Sam did not receive some of his shots for diseases like chickenpox.

He was growing up to be very happy and very healthy. He was in the 90% rank of kids of his age in both weight and height. During his first 2 and ½ years of age, he never had any serious illness other than a simple cold on two occasions and recovered from them rapidly. At age 2 years and 8 months Sam developed a very serious illness.

The Early Onset Symptoms Of Sam's Illness:

My wife opened the door of the house and stood in the doorway carrying our son Sam in her arms. I was gardening in front of our house in the rose garden. She had a worried look on her face and a nervous tremor in her voice. She said, "Sam had four bowel movements so far this morning and his stool was loose and dark brown." My mouth dried out instantly, my eyes were fixed on Sam and my mind was scrambled with numerous thoughts traveling at high speed. I remained motionless in the flower bed for a moment. Sam was our first boy and was only 2 years and 8 months old. It was mid-morning on Sunday, October 20, 1996, a sunny day with a nice soft cool breeze in Starkville, Mississippi. My wife added, "Four days ago, he started to have gas and 2 days later, he started to have frequent bowel movements."

We decided to wait until the following day, which was Monday. However, during the next three hours, Sam had three additional bowel movements. We decided to take him to a doctor at the local emergency hospital. Following a complete physical examination, the doctor ordered some routine, basic blood and stool tests which were done at the hospital. Within an hour, the doctor informed us that Sam had a stomach flu virus and that there was nothing to worry about. He added, "We see this every day during this season and it should disappear in a couple of days." The doctor recommended giving Sam some Pepto-Bismol by mouth and sent us home.

Sam's Illness Warning Messages:
A stomach flu virus? No. A missed diagnosis.

Following our visit to the local ER, we were pleased to hear it was a simple stomach flu virus and that there was nothing major to be concerned about. However, our relief did not last for long. On the contrary, our worries started to intensify gradually. Sam's condition did not improve during the following days as the doctor expected. The frequency of his bowel movements increased steadily from about 10 to more than 20 a day within five days after our visit to the doctor. The appearance of his stool became very worrisome. Blood mixed with mucus became clearly visible in his stool. We rushed Sam to his regular pediatrician. He immediately consulted Dr. P., a specialist in Jackson, Mississippi. We were scheduled to see Dr. P. on Wednesday October 30, 1996 at 12:30 PM.

Visiting The Specialist And Our First Horrible Experience:

Learn from our experience and do your best to choose the right doctor for your loved one with ulcerative colitis.

Both my wife and I drove our son to see the specialist in Jackson, Mississippi. Following a brief physical examination and listening to our observations about his condition, the doctor suspected that Sam had colitis (inflammation of the colon).

He recommended an endoscopic examination of the colon (colonoscopy). To put it very mildly, this procedure was the most horrifying experience for all of us, but particularly for our boy, who was under 3 years old.

The endoscope had a long flexible hose-like tube that was inserted into the little boy's rectum. Sam instantly started screaming and struggling violently. I was holding his arms very tightly, while my wife was holding his head to stop him from banging it on the table. A nurse was holding his legs. The pain was excruciating. Sam was struggling so violently that we all lost control of him. The procedure was performed without any anesthesia or even simple sedation. After our failed efforts to hold our son still, the doctor suggested wrapping him with a bed sheet to limit his struggling and to have a better control on him.

The endoscope tube that was inserted into the rectum had a miniature camera and a light source on its tip so the doctor could view the lining of the colon on a video monitor. The time passed by extremely slowly considering the crying and the pain our son was experiencing, along with our anxious concerns. Suddenly, our thoughts and emotions were distracted when the doctor said, "Here we go." We instantly stared at the television screen to see what the doctor had found. A sense of relief leaked in his voice as if he found what he was looking for in Sam's colon. Apparently what he found confirmed his suspicion and answered the dilemma.

After seconds of dead silence, Dr. P. started describing his findings on the monitor, "Here, we are looking at the lining of a normal colon which is glistening pink-red. Here, you see stool mixed with mucus in large amounts and these dark masses in the lumen of the colon are clotted blood. This bright red fluid is fresh blood. These round areas on lining of the colon are ulcers. They have an irregular, round edge and rough eroded surface. These ulcers are the source of bleeding," he added. The doctor pinched pieces of the lining of the colon where the ulcers were and submitted them to the laboratory for examination under the microscope for abnormalities that were not able to be seen by the naked eye.

The endoscope tube was pulled out. Sam was relieved, and gradually but very slowly stopped crying and fell into deep sleep from exhaustion. All of this took place on a table in a room at the back of the doctor office. It was like slow torture for Sam and his parents. My wife and I were literally numb, speechless, and motionless fearing the seriousness of our son's illness. It was a nerve wrecking experience that leaves me scarred with the horrible memory.

Sam's First Hospitalization:
Why was hospitalization needed?

Based on these colonoscopy findings, Sam was admitted right away to the hospital, which was connected to the doctor's office. This was his first hospitalization. He received a full and complete physical examination again by the intern doctor. His temperature, pulse, heart, and lungs were normal. He was 43 inches in length and weighed 38 pounds, a well-nourished and well-developed white male. Everything else was unremarkable, the doctor noted in the chart.

Several blood and stool samples were taken from Sam upon admission for various laboratory tests. Blood drawing and testing became almost an everyday routine procedure during his stay in the hospital. They were requesting all possible tests they could think of to find the underlying cause of the ulcers in his colon.

His initial blood values were within normal limits. All tests performed on his stool, including checking for various parasites and cultures for bacteria were negative (normal). In other words, no evidence of infection with harmful bacteria was found. The cause of the ulcers in his colon remained obscure.

Radiographs and CT scans of the abdomen were also performed on the following days and revealed no additional information about his gut's damages or further abnormalities elsewhere in his abdomen. Like blood and stool testing, various abdominal imaging techniques and biopsies became routine procedures for this young boy for years.

How Was Sam's Illness Initially Diagnosed And Treated?

What was the most useful procedure to confirm Sam's ulcerative colitis?

Although the history of frequent bouts of diarrhea with blood and mucus raise the suspicion that Sam had colitis, the colonoscopy and biopsy examinations were the two most useful tests that offer the initial confirmation of colitis. The cause of his colitis, whether it was infectious colitis caused by germs or ulcerative colitis involving the immune system, remained unclear for long time. It was gradually yet slowly defined to be UC.

Examination of the pinched tissue samples taken from the colon lining under the microscope (biopsy) revealed that Sam had colitis most likely compatible with infection due to bacteria or virus. But another disease entity known as ulcerative colitis remained a possibility, the doctor declared.

During the first seven days of hospitalization, Sam was given two types of antibiotics: Flagyl and Ciprofloxacin by mouth, pending the result of stool testing to identify the possible germs causing his illness. However, no harmful germs were identified and all stool and blood tests revealed no infection. Moreover, the antibiotics did not stop the bleeding. Therefore, Dr. P. started to lean towards the possibility that Sam had ulcerative colitis.

The exact cause of ulcerative colitis remains unknown. The disease is currently classified as an autoimmune illness. In simple terms, it is presumed that there is some defect in the control switch of the immune regulator of the intestine in people with UC. The regulator is out of control for some unknown reason and does not turn off when it supposed to. In people with UC, the immune system overreacts to foreign substances that normally would not evoke such an extreme response. This adverse overreaction incites an influx of inflammatory cells and chemicals into the intestine that results in injuries to the lining of the intestine. The immune system which normally protects the lining of the intestine is overreacting for some unknown reason, and consequently causes severe injuries in the lining of the intestine called "self-mutilation".

Dr. P. initiated medication with steroids to calm down the immune system and reduce the inflammation. Sam started receiving prednisone by mouth on November 6, 1996, the eighth day of hospitalization. The frequency of his bowel movements started to decrease noticeably during the following days. He also had much less blood in his stool. It seemed that the prednisone did the trick and brought his symptoms into remission.

Sam remained stable and was discharged from the hospital on November 11, 1996 with the plan to continue the prednisone and Flagyl at home. He was also taking an iron supplement because he lost significant amounts of his blood. His hematocrit (a measure of red blood cell volume) was 33 on day of admission and was 26.7 on the day of discharge. Normal hematocrit value is approximately 45.

Throughout his hospital stay, Sam maintained a good appetite and appeared well and healthy except for the bloody mucoid stool. He remained playful during the day and slept well at night.

It was a long 13 day stay at the hospital but we were so pleased to have our son's health problem under control.

At home, Sam continued to receive his medications as instructed. He maintained his high level of activity and a good appetite. The frequency of his bowel movements dropped from about 20 a day shortly after the start of his illness, to about 5 a day after putting him on prednisone. This gradually decreased to once or twice a day approximately 4 weeks following the initial prednisone medication. He had his first formed stool with no apparent blood on December 7, 1996, a month after initial treatment with prednisone. However, Sam remained very pale due to blood loss even though he continued receiving the liquid iron which he hated most among his medications because of its bad smell and quivering taste.

Follow-up visits with Dr. P. in Jackson, Mississippi were made on a weekly basis. In all visits, Sam's physical examination and blood tests revealed no remarkable findings except that he was slightly anemic and had low iron values. Because Sam had such deep red hair, we joked with him that his hair was hiding all of the iron that we had been giving him. On December 3, 1996, a second endoscopic examination of the colon was performed by Dr. P., and tissue samples (biopsies) were also taken from the lining of his colon. We were pleased to learn that Sam had no more visible ulcers in his colon. Also, we were told that the tissue samples examined under the microscope were normal.

Sam's First Flare Up- What Happened And Why?

Is there any medication that cures ulcerative colitis?

After his discharge from the hospital on November 11, 1996, Sam, who weighed 38 pounds at that time, continued to take 30 mg prednisone tablets by mouth once a day. We were happy to see him doing fine. On January 22, 1997, Dr. P. recommended to taper the dose of prednisone gradually. Forty days later, and while we were still tapering the dose of prednisone, Sam started bleeding on March 3, 1997. I was attending a professional meeting in California and had to cancel my trip and to come back home to Mississippi. Because Sam was attached to me, I suspected at first that the stress of my absence caused his relapse. However, this observation was not confirmed following my future traveling without him. Dr. P. recommended by phone that we should put him back on 30 mg prednisone once a day, the maximum allowed dose of prednisone for his weight.

Sam was taking 15 mg prednisone tablet by mouth once daily when the bleeding started. Prednisone is not meant to be for long term use because of its side effects and it should have been backed up by another medication, such as one of the aminosalicylates, to maintain the remission status while tapering the prednisone. Dr. P. did not recommend that and perhaps he thought that he had cured Sam's UC.

Sam's Colitis Started Getting Aggressive: *Does ulcerative colitis change its course?*

We doubled the dose of prednisone after Sam's first flare up but this time the bleeding did not stop. On the contrary, Sam's health deteriorated more day after day and more concerning signs developed. The disease started to reflect its real stubborn and aggressive nature for the first time. Sam started to complain about abdominal pain due to the erupting ulcers in his gut, about feeling cold due to being anemic, and he began to sleep more often for longer hours. He gradually stopped eating and drinking including his milk. He was very pale. Occasionally, he had sweating episodes commonly seen in patients taking prednisone. We were saddened and concerned, to say the least by these developments. I called Dr. P. and scheduled a visit with him.

I took my son to see Dr. P. early in the morning on April 2, 1997, which happened to be my birthday. We lived in Starkville, Mississippi, about a 2 ½ hour drive from Jackson, Mississippi where Dr. P. was located.

Following a brief physical examination of my son, the doctor ordered some blood tests, as usual, and informed me that he would call me with the results.

Apparently, Sam's complaints of abdominal pain, feeling cold, not eating or drinking, being very pale, and having cold hands and feet were not enough to alert Dr. P. to think twice about what was going on or to take a more aggressive action. So I drove my son back home. As I was parking the car at home, my wife came out to tell me that Dr. P. called and wanted to hospitalize Sam. The blood tests revealed that Sam was dangerously anemic. His hematocrit (a measure of blood volume) was 14 versus the normal 45. It was a life threatening level.

Sam's Second Hospitalization:
Out of the hospital and back again

On that same day, April 2, 1997, I drove Sam back to Jackson, Mississippi. Sam was very sick, and I was tired after driving more than 10 hours back and forth from home to Jackson. Sam was hospitalized at 9:30 that night. He was given 2 units of blood (total of 350 ml) throughout the night. His color came back to normal following the transfusion and he stopped complaining of being cold. Prior to the transfusion, he was breathing very fast. His heart was pounding very rapidly at a rate of 180 per minute, trying to supply oxygen to the body with a small volume of blood. This was a life threatening situation which could have caused heart fatigue and subsequent failure. His heart rate trended down to the low 100's per minute after the transfusion. This was Sam's first blood transfusion and his second hospitalization. Sam's hematocrit jumped from 14 to 25.6 after the blood transfusion.

Five days passed following the hospitalization, with not much improvement noted in terms of frequency of bowel movements. On top of this, he continued to bleed. His appetite did not improve. He was not eating or drinking at all. The nurse informed me that the doctor had ordered the placement of an intravenous line the following day if Sam continued not to drink. On the sixth day after being hospitalized, they started to give him nutrients and fluid intravenously. His hand started to swell due to misplacement of the needle in the vein so they switched the intravenous line to the other hand. Can you imagine what this 3 year old boy was going through and the heart wrenching feelings we were experiencing?

The frequency of bowel movements increased to 10 times a day and his stool was mixed with mucus and blood. He became restless and weak. He was complaining of abdominal cramps and pain, and was constantly crying and holding his stomach.

He also started to have an uncomfortable straining and an urge to defecate but no stool came out. These symptoms are called "tenesmus" and are caused by the sensation of incomplete emptying of intestine. The intestinal ulcers and inflammation irritate the intestinal nerves in such a way that gives him a burning sensation and a feeling that there was stool present and ready to be evacuated, when in actuality, there was none. Instead, blood and mucus with gas come out and he felt momentarily relieved. These straining episodes became gradually more frequent and more intense.

For the first time, Sam started making a high pitched screaming noise while straining to defecate. He was losing drops of blood slowly but continuously. His hematocrit dropped again to 21 and was transfused once more on April 7, 1996 with 2 units of blood.

He developed a fever during his stay at the hospital which spiked to 102° F. He also started to vomit every time an oral medication was given to him. For this reason, they quit giving him medications. They eliminated any and all pain medication or antibiotics by mouth or any other routes.

I stayed with my son at the hospital for this entire period, during both hospitalizations in October 1996 and April 1997. I lived every moment of the pain my son was going through. I left my job, home, and family behind. To describe my emotions while hearing my son suffering and screaming in pain is beyond what any words can describe. I was terrified as the father of this baby. I could feel the sufferings my boy was going through. I was completely devastated to watch him.

It Was About Time For A Second Opinion:
No one will be dismayed by asking experts for the right direction.

It was apparent that prednisone was not enough by itself to stop the bleeding this time and that a stronger medication was needed. On April 7, 1997 I expressed my concerns to Dr. P. about my son's ongoing bleeding, pain, and sufferings. He kept telling me to be patient, and that it would take time for the prednisone to control the problem. He was reluctant to try stronger medications.

So I decided to seek out a second medical opinion. I discussed this idea with my wife and contacted the Crohn's & Colitis Foundation of America. They recommended talking to Dr. W. in Alabama. I called Dr. W. right away and discussed with him my son's medical history, the medications given to him, and his current status. He suggested modifying his medication plan such as dividing the prednisone dose and giving it two times a day instead of once. Also, the medications that caused him to gag could be given in a liquid form and this would not cause gagging like the pill did. Moreover, the iron supplement, antibiotics, and pain medications could also be given intravenously instead of by mouth. Finally, if prednisone did not stop the bleeding, stronger medications such as cyclosporine could be tried.

Unlike Dr. P., Dr. W. had seen and treated this illness in young children of Sam's age. I expressed to Dr. W. my desire to move to Alabama and he agreed to take my son as his patient. On April 7, 1997, I politely related these suggestions regarding the medication plan to Dr. P. but he was reluctant to use cyclosporine because of its potential side effects. However, Dr. P. approved the transfer to Alabama. I drove Sam from Jackson, Mississippi to Alabama early in the morning on April 8, 1997, and Sam was hospitalized upon our arrival.

On The Road To Alabama: Seeking Out Of State Help

This was our first out of state move to seek help for my son and his third hospitalization. Following admission on April 8, 1997, Sam received a complete physical examination, more blood and stool tests, abdominal radiographs and CT scan.

He was hooked up to an intravenous set and received fluids and was transfused with 1 unit of blood. This was his third transfusion of blood within a month. On the third day after admission, an endoscopic examination of his colon (colonoscopy) was performed to see the extent of damage. More tissue samples of the intestinal lining were taken for examination under the microscope. Unlike the horrifying experience we had before, the colonoscopy procedure this time was without any struggling or suffering because it was performed under general anesthesia.

The endoscopic examination revealed extensive and diffuse ulceration throughout the lining of his colon. These ulcers were the source of the bleeding. Sam was transfused again for the fourth time within a month with 200 ml blood on April 12, 1997.

Sam Responded To A Modified Medical Plan:

As discussed on the phone, doctors in Alabama would initially attempt to stabilize Sam by modifying the plan of medication rather than changing the type of medications.

They would give him the same amount of daily allowance of prednisone but they administered half of it in the morning and the other half in the evening. Dividing the dose of prednisone and administering it every 12 hours versus once every 24 hours was an attempt to maintain the steroid activity in the body throughout the day. This was due to the duration of steroid activity in the body being uncertain; therefore it may not last for 24 hours.

Also, the medications were ordered to be given intravenously rather than by mouth to avoid his gagging reflex. In addition, intravenous medications would be available for action faster than the oral route. Sam started to show slow, but progressive improvements on this plan. Sam had his first normal appearing stool without any apparent blood 12 days later on April 20, 1997.

As If The Colitis Complications Weren't Enough, Nurses Can Sometimes Chip In

On April 20, 1997, Sam appeared healthy, stable, playful, and had an excellent appetite. Above all, he had normal stool in both appearance and frequency. The plan was to start giving his medications by mouth instead of intravenously with the hope that we could return home 3 to 4 days later. The only medication that was left to be given intravenously was the prednisone (solu-medrol).

Just when we thought we had solved the problem, unexpectedly, Sam developed severe abdominal pain and a fever of 101° F on April 21, 1997. He stopped eating. The combination of fever and pain was alarming and very serious. Fever usually indicates severe disease and/or a serious complication in ulcerative colitis patients, such as an abscess in the abdomen. Doctors were concerned that Sam might have developed a perforation in his colon. Such perforation occurs when an ulcer progresses deep into the wall of the bowel and finally ruptures. This would result in an escape of waste into the abdomen causing pain and fever.

Right away, several tests were performed with urgency to exclude or confirm the existence of a hole in his intestine. At first, X-rays, ultrasound, and CT scan of the abdomen were performed one procedure after another. Then X-rays with barium were taken. Several radiographs were taken following the intake of the milky or chalky barium by mouth. No escaped barium outside the intestinal tract was noticed, which meant there was no hole in his intestine.

At that point, doctors started to suspect that the intravenous catheter was contaminated and became a source of infection in his blood and caused the fever. The intravenous catheter was removed and a new one was inserted. The removed catheter was submitted for culture of contaminating bacteria. Sam's temperature dropped to normal on the second day following removal of the old intravenous catheter and of the antibiotic administration.

The culture results confirmed the catheter was contaminated with bacteria commonly inhabiting the skin of humans (staphylococci). The catheter gets contaminated when nurses touch the catheter around its entrance into the vein without being careful about sterility. The catheter was routinely checked daily by nurses to make sure it was in place, not leaking, and to make sure that skin under the tapes and dressings holding the catheter was fine.

The Horrific Mistake And The Second Major Flare Up In Alabama:

Guess what happens when there are too many chefs in the kitchen?

During his one month hospital stay in Alabama, Sam was seen by at least five doctors and several nurses. Some saw him in the morning and others in the evening. Some doctors took days off, including the main doctor in charge of Sam, as new ones came in. I was the only permanent person with my son. Therefore, I started to hear contradicting opinions from various doctors and see variations in the medication plan, adding and deleting medicines according to the opinion that the attending doctor dictates. Then, these additions and deletions were reversed by the main doctor in charge when she came back on duty. In spite of all of this mess, I remained pleased, since my son was progressing very well. However, the price of having "too many cooks in the kitchen" was paid for rather tragically.

During the scheduled last 4 days of our stay (April 21 to 24, 1997) at the hospital in Alabama, Sam was receiving all of his medications by mouth except the steroid solu-medrol which was being given intravenously. This was a four-day-trial period to ensure that Sam would not vomit if given medications by mouth and would not relapse.

On the morning of April 24, 1997, the day we were supposed to go home, Sam had a strong smelling bowel movement with a large amount of blood and mucus. I immediately fell into shock. My entire body was numb and my heart was frozen. I felt like all of my systems failed to function, including my breathing and heart. He had four additional similar frightening bowel movements later that morning. Sam had never had such a large amount of blood and mucus in his stool while being in this hospital because he had been on prednisone since he was discharged from the hospital in Jackson, Mississippi. Dr. B. the primary doctor in charge froze speechless when she saw the stool. What happened? Why did he flare up? Sadness could be sensed among doctors and nurses on the floor. Speaking was physically difficult for me. I was crying uncontrollably and chocking with back tears. I felt hopeless.

On the same afternoon of that day, a new nurse came in to check on Sam. I saw her moving the intravenous pole out of the room. I asked, "Why are you moving the pole out?" Surprisingly, she replied "There is no need for it". When I asked her about the prednisone she said, "Prednisone has not been given for the past 4 days". My jaw dropped and my face froze. I was stunned. We checked the medical record and sure enough, she confirmed to me that prednisone had been discontinued 4 days ago.

A follow up inquiry revealed that the prednisone was not omitted by the doctor, but a nurse who committed a mistake. It was heart-wrenching to see my son had relapsed. It was a horrific tragedy to learn the relapse occurred because of a mistake made by the nurse.

Some tried to dismiss the incident, fearing its consequences, while others were honestly dismayed and regretted it. The news spread rather quickly among attending nurses and doctors and found its way to the highest level of the hospital's management.

I left my job and my family. The chair next to my son had been my bed for the past several weeks. I was going through devastating emotions, and paying thousands of dollars being an out of state patient, only to experience mistakes by nurses and a lack of leadership of doctors. My confidence and trust in doctors and nurses became seriously shaken. I was going through a crisis of confidence. Doctors who were doing their routine tours came in to see me sobbing that morning. I could not physically speak to them because I was unable to hold back tears. Instead, I was pointing to Sam's diapers which were filled with mucus and blood. They left the room with sadness realizing that Sam had flared up once again.

When they learned about the reason for the relapse, the doctors and nurses were totally dismayed and anguished. All commented that this should have never happened. Doctors and nurses apologized and comforted. I aged years in a matter of days.

At first, Dr. B., the doctor in charge of my son, did not make any comments or apology on the incident. Later, and apparently because the pressure was mounting on her and on the nurse who committed the mistake, Dr. B. finally said "I will be on the top of this incident and it will not be easy for the nurse who committed this mistake." The head nurse of the hospital, management people, and the social worker came to apologize and to comfort. "An error like this should never happen, no excuse for it," they commented. "We know this is frustrating for you. We are trying to say to you that the incident will not go unnoticed."

Some nurses brought Sam a gift. Others offered a hug. Every one apologized and offered comforting words except the nurse who committed the mistake. She offered a sad excuse. She said, "I gave Sam the prednisone but I did not write it down on chart because there was not much room on the chart." This excuse was so sad because the well-known unwritten medical law states "If it is not noted in the medical chart it did not happen." Everyone knew this.

Regardless of this fact, the nurse was not very honest. I played the detective and investigator role to uncover the facts of what had really happened and why my son had flared up. I discovered that the nurse did not give any prednisone to my son during the past four days contrary to her claims, because I found out that the pharmacy did not dispense any prednisone for Sam for four days prior to his relapse. The nurse was not telling the truth. She committed a mistake and consistently did not reveal the truth, which affected an innocent sick child because of her pride. The pharmacy explained that the doctor writes prescriptions on an order form. The nurse transfers the order to the patient's chart and copies the pharmacy to dispense the medications. In our case the nurse failed to do so and the pharmacy did not dispense prednisone for Sam.

Following this incident, Sam was moved to a room in the semi-intensive care ward where only one or two patients are assigned for each nurse so that more careful attention can be given to my son. After hours of straining and crying in pain, Sam found comfort in a teddy bear a nurse gave it to him and fell to sleep.

Tragedies Happen For A Reason:

My faith taught me that there is a reason and much to learn from the adverse events that happen to people in this life. All you need is to search for them. So I forgave myself and the nurse and allowed myself to move forward and not get stuck in the tragedy of this relapse. Looking at the flare up from a positive angle, the nurse's mistake was an opportunity to prove that Sam's colitis demands prednisone to calm down. It appears that his colitis was literally addicted to prednisone. Before this particular flare up, comments were made by doctors in Alabama that my son did not need prednisone or any other immunosuppressive medications to treat his colitis. They thought that some sort of germs were involved in Sam's illness rather than having the autoimmune ulcerative colitis. Their conclusion was solely based on interpretation of the findings in Sam's colon samples under the microscope. The findings were not the characteristic findings of UC according to their experience.

One would assume that if there was some sort of germ involved, the prednisone would have aggravated his condition rather than calmed it down because of the immunosuppression effect caused by the prednisone. But this was not what doctors in Alabama believed.

AGGRESSIVE COLITIS DEMANDS AGGRESSIVE MEDICATIONS:
The last flare up of Sam's colitis in Alabama was due to the mistake of not receiving prednisone for four days and because

of the slow response to prednisone after the first and second flare ups. This made us realize that Sam not only needed steroids to calm his immune system and to stop the rectal bleeding, but also proved that prednisone alone was not efficacious enough to attain remission quickly. A stronger medication than prednisone was clearly needed to control his illness and to stop the bleeding. It was becoming gradually more evident that Sam had a "hot colitis" which means that his immune system is violently attacking (self-mutilating) the lining of his colon.

On Wednesday April 26, 1997, two days after the erroneous flare up, Sam started receiving cyclosporine intravenously in one arm. He also started receiving the prednisone through another intravenous line in the other arm. Within one day following cyclosporine therapy, Sam started to show noticeable improvements. He became more active, playful, and retained his appetite. Sam continued receiving both cyclosporine and prednisone intravenously for 6 days until May 2, 1997. Then he was switched to cyclosporine, imuran (another immunomodulators drug), and prednisone by mouth.

Sam continued to improve while daily blood tests were performed to monitor the level of cyclosporine and other blood values. He had only one bowel movement, without any noticeable blood, on May 6, 1997. As his rectal bleeding had stopped, his blood values began to improve. He was discharged from the hospital on May 7, 1997. That was a whole 30 days of hospitalization with fluctuating emotions but at least my son was stable for a time.

Cyclosporine is a very potent suppressor of the immune system and is widely used in patients with an organ transplant to prevent rejection of the transplanted organ. Cyclosporine has many serious toxic effects which have been elaborated on "under treatment of ulcerative colitis". One of the immediate concerns is that cyclosporine has been reported to cause liver and kidney damage and subsequent failure. In addition to the daily routine blood testing that had been ongoing while Sam being hospitalized, more blood and urine tests were now added to closely evaluate his kidneys and liver and to monitor the level of cyclosporine in his blood.

At home, Sam continued to take his medications as instructed and was doing well. He was taking prednisone, cyclosporine, Imuran, Flagyl, and an iron supplement. Blood testing was performed on a weekly basis to monitor his basic blood values and to check the level of cyclosporine in his blood. Cyclosporine blood level monitoring was done only in certain laboratories and had to be sent out of state depending on availability of such laboratories. Special requirements and precautions need to be followed while mailing blood samples for cyclosporine testing. In addition, the test was very expensive and may not be covered by health insurance.

The Flare Up/Remission Cycles Of Ulcerative Colitis And The Hopeless Feeling That Medication Would Not Bring An End To This Misery:

Sam started straining and bleeding again on June 10, 1997, approximately 6 weeks after starting the cyclosporine. This time, the disease grabbed hold. Sam's symptoms progressed from cramping and diarrhea during the day, to nocturnal diarrhea with bleeding and pain. His appetite to eat and drink declined and he began to lose strength. We increased the dose of both prednisone and cyclosporine, as recommended by Dr. W. of Alabama, but this barely took the edge off. He continued to deteriorate and he was hospitalized again in Alabama on Sunday June 15, 1997, which happened to be Father's Day.

This was his third major flare up and his fourth hospitalization. We knew from prior experience that once relapsed, he would need a very aggressive medication plan and stronger drugs to stabilize him again. While his colitis was controlled with oral prednisone initially, he needed prednisone, Imuran, Pentasa, Flagyl and cyclosporine to calm it down. Following a 10-day-hospitalization, intensive care, and strong medications given intravenously, Sam was discharged from the hospital on June 25, 1997.

Doctors believed that Sam's colitis was very severe and was not responding properly to medications. Doctors recommended surgery to remove Sam's colon. I felt that such recommendation was coming eventually, but I hated to hear it. We were referred to a specialist, Dr. P., in Pennsylvania.

I started searching for a job in Pennsylvania and mailing my resume to several potential employers. At the same time, we listed our home in Mississippi for sale. A buyer made an offer and we accepted it in a heartbeat, without any negotiation or hesitation. We closed the sale and received the payment on July 15, 1997. That was 20 days after Sam was discharged from the hospital in Alabama. On the following day, July 16, 1997, all of our household goods were on a U-Haul truck and we hit the road that morning on our way to Pennsylvania. This was our second major out of state move.

On The Road To Pennsylvania: The Second Move Out Of State

We arrived in Pennsylvania on July 20, 1997. Considering the unpredictability of Sam's flare ups, we picked up a primary care physician the day after we arrived in town and visited the specialist, Dr. P., right away.

I was offered a job in a veterinary hospital minutes from Dr. P. I started my new job on September 2, 1997, the day after Labor Day. That day, Sam began to bleed again. This was his fourth flare up. So far, his relapses coincided with my birthday, Father's Day, when I went out of town, and now on my 1st day of my new job. Luckily, this time we were able to stabilize him by increasing the dose of cyclosporine according to Dr. P.'s recommendations and without hospitalization.

If It Is Not The Unpleasant Flare Up Symptoms, It Is The Ugly Side Effects Of The Medications:

After his fourth flare up, Sam continued to do well after we increased the dose of cyclosporine. He had no loose stools, no visible bleeding, no abdominal pain, and his appetite to eat and to drink remained normal. It seemed that his colitis had finally given us a break and was under control.

However, if this was not the case, it is that kind of situation. Sam was now 3 years and 7 months old. His colitis was one year old. He did not grow in height at all during the past year and he gained only 6 pounds. His poor growth in both weight and height was mostly because of his colitis and partly because of the side effects of medications, mainly the steroid. His gums were thickened because of the cyclosporine. He had hair overgrowth on his face and body because of cyclosporine and steroids and remained pale due to blood loss. He had been on cyclosporine, Pentasa, prednisone, and Imuran for over a year now. In spite of all the iron supplements that Sam was taking, his blood tests revealed low iron level. On a few occasions Sam received a bolus of iron intravenously to bring it to an acceptable level.

The Challenging Nature Of Sam's Ulcerative Colitis: Dr. P. of Pennsylvania instructed us with a plan to reduce the dose of prednisone gradually which we followed. As of November 1st 1997, Sam was no longer on prednisone but continued taking the other medications; cyclosporine, Pentasa, and Imuran. Two months after being weaned off the prednisone, Sam started in January of 1998 to have frequent bowel movements and complaints of abdominal pain. Although he was still on potent immunosuppressive medications, it was clear that Sam's colitis was getting more active after removing the prednisone from the treatment list, but the colitis was not as active as it had been previously. We continued to monitor his activities and his blood counts.

Although there was no obvious bleeding, repeated blood tests revealed low red blood cell values, indicating that he was continuously losing invisible amounts of blood in stool over time. He was hospitalized and received a blood transfusion on February 21, 1998. During this hospital stay, he was also endoscoped under general anesthesia while his esophagus, stomach, small and large intestines were examined. Tissue samples were also taken from all of these scoped organs for examination under the microscope.

No active colitis was visible on the colonoscopy. Examination of tissue samples under the microscope revealed findings that raised suspicion of food allergy as a possible cause of his colitis. Food allergy tests were performed and were negative for the food ingredients he was taking at that time. We continued to see Dr. P. in Pennsylvania for about a year and then he recommended that we see his professor Dr. R. in the state of Delaware.

On The Road To Delaware: The Third Out-Of-State Run

Sam's ulcerative colitis kept us on the run all the time. Rather than moving to Delaware we settled in Lancaster, PA because I found a job there in a small animal hospital. Lancaster, PA was about 1½ hour drive from Dr. R. in Delaware. This was the third major move and was not the best move we made. It was full of flare ups and complications.

Beware How Immunosuppressives Work:
Side effects of immunosuppressive medications

Because ulcerative colitis attacked Sam at an early age and because he was placed on immunosuppressive medications to keep him in remission, Sam did not receive some of his shots to prevent diseases like chickenpox. On August 17, 1998, Sam's friend became sick with chickenpox. We were very concerned about Sam contracting chickenpox from his friend because of Sam's suppressed immune system. We took Sam to the emergency hospital that evening and he received prophylactic medications and immunization. Unfortunately this was not completely helpful. Twelve days later Sam developed the lesions of chickenpox. It started with a fever and reddish pimples on his skin of the abdomen, back, and legs. These pimples quickly progressed into blisters and then they ruptured. He started receiving acyclovir, an anti-viral medication and fortunately Sam recovered in a few days.

Two months later, Sam started to have abdominal cramps and frequent bowel movements with flecks of blood in his stool early October 1998. Laboratory tests revealed that his blood cyclosporine level was very low. Also, Sam began retake prednisone after he ceased to take it for one year. The dose of cyclosporine was also increased per doctor recommendation and the bleeding seemed to stop shortly after that. We learned that absorption of cyclosporine from the intestine is very erratic and unpredictable. In other words, blood levels of cyclosporine fluctuate. For this reason, we checked the blood cyclosporine level almost every two weeks to make sure acceptable levels are maintained.

In late October 1998, Sam developed an extremely painful skin rash with blisters on various parts of his body and was hospitalized with diagnosis of herpes zoster, commonly known as shingles. The initial infection with chickenpox virus caused this acute short-lived illness. Once an episode of chickenpox had resolved, the virus was not completely eliminated from the body but stayed hiding in a dormant phase and could go on to cause shingles many years after the initial infection. The blisters ruptured and left crusty lesions and scars. Some scars are still visible on his skin to this day. Blood tests revealed that the cyclosporine level was very high. Sam developed zoster because he was severely immunosuppressed due to high level of cyclosporine, in addition to the prednisone and imuran; all of which are immunosuppressive drugs. Sam recovered shortly after correcting the level of cyclosporine and was released from the hospital in Delaware.

The original plan of putting Sam on cyclosporine was only intended for 6 months. We planned to also to take him off prednisone and maintain him on a milder medication such as Pentasa. That plan was never possible because he flared up once the prednisone dose was lowered or the level of cyclosporine in his blood dropped. Sam had been on cyclosporine, Imuran, and Pentasa for 18 months and he still continued on prednisone. Although these medications seemed to calm down his colitis, their toxic effects can be very serious and some of these negative effects had already been seen in Sam. Doctors in Delaware discussed with us the alternative approach to save Sam from his misery, which predictably was surgery to remove his large intestine. For this reason we were recommended to go to California.

On The Road Again: Moving To California, The Final Destination

We were on the run during the past three years looking for the doctor who could magically cure our son. In June 26, 1999, we packed our belongings and left Pennsylvania for California. This was our fourth out-of-state move.

Signs Of Feeling Comfortable With Your Doctor:

We selected a primary care physician and met the specialist Dr. M. in northern California. She was a pediatrician who dealt with colitis in children on a regular basis. She was easy to talk to and listened very well. We had no feelings of being rushed. On top of that, she talked with an assuring voice and confidence, "I will find out for you what Sam's problem is." In our first visit, Dr. M. listened to our observations carefully. We immediately felt very comfortable with Dr. M. As a matter of fact, we trusted Dr. M. from our first visit.

Here We Go Again: Testing, Testing, And More

So far, all of the specialists we visited in the various states followed the same accustomed steps. They listen to us, they did a thorough examination on Sam, and then they recommended various tests. Dr. M. was not the exception. She referred Sam to see a heart specialist because of his anemia and to see an eye specialist to evaluate his vision because of the toxic effects of the medications he had been on for so long.

In addition, Dr. M. requested and reviewed records of all previous hospitalization in Mississippi, Pennsylvania, and Delaware. She also requested the actual preparations of all tissues biopsies sampled from Sam that were taken at the previous hospitals. Dr. M. wanted to view these tissues with her colleagues to have a clear idea of what was going on. Basically, she wanted to evaluate the progression of his illness over the past three years. She also ordered stool cultures, urine tests and various blood tests to check Sam's current blood values, medications levels, and vital organs functions. It was easy to say and write all these things, but living through them was a different story.

She also requested a blood test to differentiate between ulcerative colitis and Crohn's disease. Abdominal X-rays with and without barium along with CT scan of the abdomen were also ordered. Dr. M. also hospitalized Sam for two days to perform endoscopy of the esophagus, stomach, and small intestine, as well as a colonoscopy under general anesthesia. She took samples of tissues from the various scoped organs for microscopic examination. This was Sam's fifth endoscopic examination and biopsy since the start of his illness and his sixth hospitalization.

Intestinal Motility Test:

Examination of tissue samples under the microscope in California revealed some local nerve damage which raised concerns about the possibility that Sam had a slower than normal colon motility (contraction) in addition to ulcerative colitis. Dr. M. referred us to Dr. H. in southern California to evaluate motility of the colon.

Sam was hospitalized on June 18, 2000 for three days to perform this procedure. The results revealed that Sam had poor motility and nerve responses in his colon. This explained the frequent stool impactions seen in Sam's colon during the past 3 years. Poor motility of the colon was due to injury of the nerves supplying the colon.

The nerve problem could be a birth defect, damage caused by ulcerative colitis, a side effect of cyclosporine, or the nerves were mechanically overstretched due to retention of stool in the colon which caused it to be greatly distended. The lining of the colon was also examined by Dr. H. and the colitis was described as being inactive. Surgery was recommended by Dr. H. to remove his colon because of its poor motility and the history of frequent relapses of ulcerative colitis.

Hearing What You Do Not Like To Hear From Your Doctor – "Surgery"

When we moved to California, Sam was 5 years and 8 months old. He had just started kindergarten. His weight was 49 pounds and his height was still 43 inches. During the past three years, he gained only 11 pounds. He never grew in height at all. At birth, he was in the 90th percentile for both height and weight and he was now in the 25th percentile for height and 75th percentile for weight. In spite of this, he remained well- nourished and very bright, even though he was taking several seriously toxic medications.

Endoscopic examination performed by Dr. M. confirmed that Sam's colitis was inactive and under control. Stool cultures and various other tests revealed no harmful bacteria involved in his colitis. Blood tests revealed that he was mildly anemic. Unfortunately no definitive answer was obtained from the blood tests performed to differentiate between ulcerative colitis and Crohn's disease. The cloud remained hanging around Sam's definitive diagnosis. The urine tests revealed no significant findings. The heart specialist detected a low grade heart murmur and attributed its cause to the anemia. Sam's eyes were okay.

Since the last major flare-up about two years ago, in June of 1997, Sam had been doing well. His colitis seemed to be under control, while being on several immunosuppressants. Occasional abdominal pain or flecks of blood were seen in stool but were corrected by adjusting the dose of his medications. His appetite remained healthy. He was hospitalized a couple of times but not because of his colitis. On October 5, 1999, he was hospitalized for fever associated with cold and coughing. His cough was persistent and made him gag and throw up, causing him to become dehydrated. He responded well to the fluid therapy and antibiotics and was discharged 2 days later. Another hospitalization took place on April 16, 2000 because Sam developed a fever for an unknown reason. Again, he responded well to fluid therapy and antibiotics and was discharged three days later. Whenever he developed a fever, Sam would be hospitalized and subjected to extensive blood tests, cultures of stool and urine, radiographs, CT scans, and many other tests to rule out abdominal abscess associated with perforation of the intestine.

Even though Sam's colitis had been under control for a while, Dr. M. strongly recommended against him remaining on several immunosuppressive medications for this long. She stated some of these medications are very potent immunosuppressants with very serious toxic effects. Sam had facial and body hair overgrowth, thickened gums, a puffed up face (moon face) and above all, he had poor growth in both weight and height. He never grew an inch since starting on the steroids 3 years ago. Also, his immune defense ability was impaired significantly due to these medications. Sam contracted chickenpox from contact with his friend and then shingles while he was having severe immunosuppression because of these medications.

The combination of the toxic side effects of medications and the lack of perfect response to medical therapy made Sam a perfect candidate for surgery. In our visit of August 17, 2000, Dr. M. recommended surgery for Sam to remove his colon. He was anemic and his other blood values were not healthy. "No medication is going to stop this misery" Dr. M. said. "Sam will have a better life after surgery. Most people who had this surgery had wished they have done it 10 years earlier." she added.

The ball was in our court now and the pressure to make the decision of whether to go for surgery or not was mounting. We, the parents, were now facing a very serious challenge to cut or not to cut. Once the colon was removed, it would be gone forever. What were we going to tell our son in the future if surgery did not cure his illness?

Making A Definitive Diagnosis Was A Real Challenge We Faced With Sam's Illness

Diagnosis went from tragic to controversial

From the start and continuing for years, the most challenging issue doctors faced was making a definitive diagnosis of my son's illness. The challenge facing us was to consent to surgery. Although samples of the lining of his intestine were taken on several occasions, various doctors were observing different findings under the microscope and perhaps interpreting them differently. Some features suggested that Sam had the autoimmune ulcerative colitis. Other features suggested that Sam had colitis caused by infection with germs such as bacteria or viruses. However, no harmful germs were identified in spite of the several attempts that were made. Furthermore, broad spectrum antibiotics did not stop the bleeding or attain remission or make any change in his status. Lack of response to various antibiotics may possibly exclude the possibility that his colitis was caused by bacteria. Also, no evidence of infections with viruses was ever found.

In spite of these facts, some doubts, even though very slim, remained hanging around the possible involvement of a germ in Sam's colitis. Doctors remained suspicious about the existence of a mysterious germ that they had not yet been successful in identifying. They continued their efforts in searching for these germs every time Sam flared up and was hospitalized.

Changes in tissue samples taken in Mississippi were interpreted as compatible with colitis that was caused by infection with bacteria or viruses. The second set of tissue samples taken in Mississippi were interpreted as normal. When these tissues were reviewed by doctors in California, they interpreted them differently. They considered changes in the first set of tissues as an early ulcerative colitis and changes in the second set as chronic colitis and not normal. Examination of tissue samples taken from Sam in Pennsylvania revealed findings that raised the suspicion of food allergy as a possible cause of his colitis. This was further investigated by doctors in Delaware. However, doctors in California considered these features as normal when they reviewed the same tissue preparations.

Based on tissue findings, doctors in Alabama were uncertain if prednisone was necessary for Sam. On the contrary, they suspected that prednisone might even have harmed him. As a matter of fact, they were thinking of taking him off prednisone, but they were not absolutely sure that this would be the right move.

A lot of discussions and consultations were ongoing among doctors regarding Sam's illness. Although Sam was making good progress following the addition of prednisone to his medical plan, Sam was receiving several other medications at the same time. It was not clear as to which medication was making the difference. I could see that all attending doctors were having a serious dilemma in making the right choices of medication and in particular the steroids, because of lack of an accurate and definitive diagnosis. Long term use of steroids can have negative effects on the body.

Another serious and very challenging disease that needed to be distinguished from ulcerative colitis was Crohn's disease. The significance of telling these two diseases apart was fundamentally critical if one has to consider the surgical treatment. In ulcerative colitis, the inflammation is confined to the colon and therefore surgical removal of the colon is basically a cure of ulcerative colitis. In Crohn's disease, the inflammation may affect any part of the gastrointestinal tract, from the mouth to the anus. Therefore, surgical removal of the colon as recommended for my son would not be a cure of his illness if it turned out to be Crohn's disease. Crohn's disease can recur after surgery in the remaining parts of the gastrointestinal tract. A diagnosis of Crohn's disease has been confirmed in some patients thought originally to be suffering from UC.

Unfortunately, no definitive answer was obtained from the blood tests used to differentiate ulcerative colitis from Crohn's disease. As a matter of fact, results of this blood test were negative. In other words, Sam had neither ulcerative colitis nor Crohn's disease. This added more clouds around Sam's definitive diagnosis. The test was repeated three times while being in care of doctors in Alabama, Delaware, and California. All revealed the same negative results. However, I was told that the test may give negative results under certain circumstances, such as when the disease was in remission.

Examination of tissue samples taken in California also raised concerns about the possibility that Sam has a slower than normal colon motility in addition to his ulcerative colitis. Other specialists concluded that the slow bowel movement that Sam had was secondary to the colitis, rather than primary nerve damage. They also raised concerns based on features seen in the tissues that Crohn's disease could not be entirely excluded, although no definitive evidence of Crohn's disease was seen.

To the doctors and specialists, my son's illness was a real dilemma. To me, his illness was a nightmare as one can obviously imagine.

CHAPTER 3

Should we or should we not Cut? A Serious Dilemma Facing Patients and their Caregivers Alike

WE REALIZED THAT SAM'S COLON was bad and we understood that Sam was taking serious medications but to approve colon removal was beyond these realizations.

MAKING THE TOUGH DECISION ABOUT SURGERY, MY BELIEF IN G-D AND THE POWER OF PRAYERS:

"*Oh, G-D, PLEASE HELP ME,*" my young boy screamed with a high pitched crying voice one evening, while having unbearable pain from abdominal cramps. I started crying instantly when I heard him saying this. This child was begging G-d to help him. An innocent 5- year-old-child was crying in pain and desperately begging no one else but the Almighty G-d, his creator, to help him. He did not say, "Oh, Dad, please help me." He did not say, "Oh, Doctor, please help me." He asked G-d to please help him. Have you ever had a situation where your little child is crying and begging you for something? How does that make you feel? Would not you respond and satisfy the child? Why does G-d not respond to this child's prayers? Why does G-d not respond to the prayers of his parents? Why did G-d allow this to happen in the first place? What did this child do to deserve all this suffering?

It was very painful to describe what was going on with my son. To watch him and feel his suffering and emotions and what I was going through was beyond what words could describe. I was with my son all of the time and lived through his sufferings, moment by moment.

I never lost faith in G-d. I kept praying day and night; early mornings, in the middle of nights, during the day, and at any time. I prostrated to G-d and begged Him to cure Sam. As the days went by with no response, I started to cry in my prayers and begged G-d for His mercy. Sometimes I screamed in my prayers in desperate need.

I kept talking about my son's problem with religious people of various faiths: Muslims, Christians, Jews, whenever and wherever I met them at work, in the house of G-d, and in social meetings. I was so desperate. People of various religious beliefs started to pray for my son in mass and individually. As

Sam's illness duration prolonged and extended over the years, my prayers intensified accordingly.

I sincerely believed in G-d and strongly believed in the power of prayers. G-d's promised in the Qur'an, Torah, and the Bible "Call upon me and I shall respond." His Almighty promise is very clear, assuring, and without any ambiguity. There are no strings attached to His promise except to ask for His mercy. There are no "but's", "if's", "and's", or any other terms and conditions. "Call upon me and I shall respond," period. So I continued to sincerely call upon Him but I saw no response. Because of the lack of response, stray ideas and thoughts began to cross my mind over time. I started to think that maybe I am not a true, honest, or sincere believer in Him. Maybe I am even not a good person in the eyes of G-d. This is why He is not responding to my calls. I talked to religious people of various beliefs about this specific verse "Call upon me and I shall respond." Their answer was universally the same. "We do not know why G-d does not respond to our prayers sometimes." One priest explained to me that although G-d is truthful in His promise to respond, G-d did not specify in that verse as to when He will respond. I found this answer rather amusing because I wanted G-d to respond now. I wanted my son to be cured yesterday. I am a human being. I have no more patience. My son was being ravaged by ulcerative colitis and tortured by excruciating pain. How can I or any other parent have patience in such situations?

Other ideas crossed my mind. Is G-d punishing or testing my faith in him? Is this why He is not responding? But if so, why is this child paying the price? What did my two year old boy do to deserve all this?

I intensely thought about the lack of response to my prayers from the Almighty G-d. Another weird thought crossed my mind. I had heard of cruel rulers in some overseas countries who enjoy watching opposing members being tortured. I heard of dictators in some countries who enjoy their meals and drinks while watching people being tortured upon their orders. I am by no mean comparing G-d to these psychopathic criminals. G-d is the most merciful. I believe that G-d sees and hears everything that we do and say. He is omniscient. He is everywhere. He is watching us. He is watching my son crying in excruciating pain. He is hearing me cry and beg for His mercy. Why does not He respond? Is G-d enjoying our torture? Heaven forbid, I am sure He is not. But I was confused, and may be in a state of hallucination.

I talked to people about my son and I could see how very sad and sorry they expressed themselves. Some of them even cried with me because I got emotional and cry every time I talked about my son's suffering just like now as I am writing these words. People promised to pray and to ask their friends and families to pray as well. If people were so kind, where is G-d's mercy? When was He going to shower my son and his family with His mercy?

As time went by and the suffering continued, new strange thoughts crossed my mind. I believed that G-d owns everything in this world; in the skies, in the earth, what is in between them, above them, and underneath them. They were worth nothing to Him, not even a penny. Now if I were to approach any person and beg him for a penny and explain that the penny would cure my son and bring him and his family all the happiness back they lost, would not you think that this person would give me the penny? I would think even a totally broke homeless person would happily offer me the penny under these circumstances. To G-d nothing is worth anything. If people could offer me a penny why did G-d not offer my son back his health, which is worth nothing to Him? He is the founder and owner of everything. He is the creator. He is the giver, not the taker. G-d has the power of having whatever He desired instantly and without saying a word. If so, why would not G-d, who is the most generous, offer my son that which he is missing in his body that caused his illness? Why would He not express His generosity to me by curing my son? I was not trying to challenge G-d or to ask Him to prove Himself to me. This was absolutely not my intention. I am only a human being and my son had been suffering for so long. Moreover, I am a strong believer in Him. My dilemma was, why does G-d not respond to my calls?

The Three Mysterious Events And The Perceived Messages:

Sam was in extreme pain and suffering. He reached rock bottom in term of his health condition and he looked very pale and thin. Literally, he looked like skin and bone. I almost reached a state of hopelessness. I sat down one day and started conversing with my Almighty. "G-d, You have given me Sam, a child with a serious illness. Thank you very much. Did I ever complain to you? Okay, maybe I did once in a while... but for the past three years, You have tested me again and again. I remained patient and faithful to You Almighty. It is Sam's flare ups that I would like to discuss with you today. They are extremely frightening and heart wrenching. I admit that I failed to become accustomed to them. One, two, three, four flares were not enough to break me? Not enough?! He was hospitalized 26 times in less than 3 years? Not enough?! He underwent general anesthesia 23 times? Not enough?! He had 5 blood transfusions? Not enough?! I abandoned my job and my family to be with him? Not enough?! The whole family has been on the run from one state to another for years? Not enough?! Hospitals became like my new residence. And you know how much I hate hospitals under these circumstances. I know, You helped me stop shaking at critical moments. Thank you very much."

"Only You G-d know the extent of damage inside his gut. And only You G-d know the extent of the damage inside my heart. G-d Almighty, You broke me! My heart (and my back). For 3 years I have been asking, begging, cajoling, and finally yelling to please heal Sam. Now G-d I beg You to please either heal him or take him. Please G-d, he is Your creature. You have created him. Please heal him or take him. I beg You G-d to take me as well. I have had enough suffering in this life. I need no more torture. I lost my last hanging fiber of strength. You know that. And now, You think this is not painful enough? Now, You have cornered me to decide by myself whether to cut his gut or not?"

The following day, after having spilled a river of tears while conversing with G-d with an overwhelming feeling of hopelessness, three unexplainable events took place. Two of them occurred on the same day, which was the 15th of August 2000, and a third on the following month on September 15, 2000. These events coincided at the same time Dr. M. recommended the surgery for my son. Our last visit with Dr. M. was on August 17, 2000, in which she said to me, "Do not leave this room without saying yes to surgery". Is this a coincidence?

EVENT #1:

On Tuesday, August 15, 2000, a client named Mari brought her cat to a veterinary hospital where I was working that day. The cat had a swollen ear because blood was trapped under the skin of the ear (blood blister). It was a self-inflicted problem caused by the cat scratching her ear due to irritation, caused by ear mites in this case. I explained to Mari that the cat needed a minor surgery, but under general anesthesia, to empty the blood and suture the ear. Mari asked if she could do the procedure herself at home. Just to make sure I understood what she had just said, I stared at Mari for a moment and rehearsed to myself what she had asked. Before I replied, Mari went on to say, "I do medical services to myself at home", as she lifted her T-shirt to show me a square piece of bandage taped on her right lower abdomen. I was shocked when she did that. "Do you want to see more?" she asked. In a state of curiosity and puzzlement, I asked what that was and she answered "I have ulcerative colitis". I immediately felt numbness in the skin of my face and head, my hair stuck up, and goose bumps developed all over my body, thinking ulcerative colitis was what my son is suffering from.

I had never met Mari before. This was not even the veterinary hospital where I regularly worked. A veterinarian colleague asked me to cover his shift that day. Is this a coincidence or does G-d have His unique ways to show me His plans? I asked Mari, "Would you please tell me more?" Without any hesitation or concerns, Mari went into detail about everything. She had already had two surgeries for her colitis.

In the first surgery, the entire large intestine (rectum, colon) were removed. The end of the remaining small intestine (ileum) was attached to a hole on the side of her lower abdomen (just above the flank area), a procedure is called ileostomy. The hole was attached to an external bag to collect waste and gas. She was having difficulties with that surgical approach. On one occasion, the bag fell off and waste scattered all over the floor to be noticed by people at a party Mari was attending. “It was a humiliating moment for me,” she said. She added “I wished I died that moment.” In addition, she was fired from her job because other employees noticed her going frequently to the bathroom to empty the bag. They raised health concerns. However, she challenged them legally based on discrimination against people with chronic illness at the workplace and she won the case. I listened to her intensely.

She went on to tell me about her second surgery in which a balloon (pouch) was made of the ileum (end of small intestine) to act as an internal reservoir and the neck of the pouch was attached to the hole in her lower abdomen. She had to siphon the waste every couple of hours to release the gas through the hole. This is what was covered with the square piece of gauze and tape that she showed me.

She continued to say, “I had several complications with these surgeries. The most serious were adhesions between adjacent loops of my intestine.” These adhesions occurred due to scar tissue forming bridges between walls of the intestine and are very common in abdominal surgeries in people. "The abdominal pain caused by these adhesions is excruciating. I am on many kinds of pills for pain, including a narcotic, but with little benefit. Every month, pockets of fluid are formed in my abdomen. Doctors drain them with big syringes and long needles, using ultrasound device as a guide to locate the sacs of fluid. These fluid filled sacs are formed every month and coincide with my monthly menstrual cycle."

I was literally astonished to hear Mari's story. This was the first time I had ever heard about these two surgical procedures for colitis and their complications. Before I tell you about the second incident which took place on the same day, let me first jump to a very similar incident.

EVENT #2:

On Friday September 15, 2000, Suzanne brought in her cat to my veterinary hospital. The cat had a history of allergies and was constantly scratching and itching herself. I said, "The best medication for the cat is steroids. However, the cat is on the heavy side and we need to be careful about her gaining more weight. Steroids would make the cat eat more and gain weight. So I will give you another medication that has no effects on appetite and weight, but may not be as effective an anti-allergy as the steroid."

Suzanne said, "Please give her the steroid. I am familiar with steroids. I take prednisone myself. I have colitis." Honestly, my tears started to flow instantly and uncontrollably as I listened to Suzanne. This is not only because I felt sorry for Suzanne, but also because of these unexplainable events of women with colitis telling me their stories. Suzanne was 42 years old when I met her. She was diagnosed with colitis at age 17. Medical treatment did not completely maintain her colitis in remission. Surgery was performed on her 5 years ago in which the colon was removed and the end of the small intestine (ileum) was connected directly to the anus, a procedure is called ileo-anal anastomosis or J-pouch, instead of to a hole in the abdomen, as in Mari's surgery. She said, "I have had diarrhea since I woke up from that surgery. Every time I eat, food goes through the other end to this day. I wear diapers all the time. For this reason, I work from home for a computer company." Without any hesitations, Suzanne taught me all what I needed to know about her colitis and her surgery, without me asking any questions. This is the third surgical approach for people with colitis. I heard it from Suzanne for the first time.

The least I would say about the stories of these two women was that I was truly and honestly puzzled. Who were these women? Why were they telling me very personal and private information? I had never met these women before. I never asked them or any of my clients to tell me about their health problems. As a matter of fact, I did not remember any other client ever telling me about their health issues other than Mari and Suzanne. Moreover, no clients have ever told me their health problems since these two incidents. They voluntarily described to me the three surgical approaches to ulcerative colitis in people, and the horrible complications associated with these surgeries. Were they angels?

Do I want my child to have a bag on his stomach to collect waste in a swimming pool and in front of other children, or to have excruciating pain from adhesions and diarrhea for the rest of his life? Does any father want these horrible complications for his child?

I settled and believed that G-d Almighty had sent me these women to deter me from electing the surgical approach for my son.

EVENT #3:

On the same day I saw Mari on August 15, 2000, a client named Karen brought in a 20 year old cat for examination. The cat had kidney insufficiency/failure. In veterinary medicine, the common elected option for the treatment of cats with kidney insufficiency included fluid therapy twice or more a week for the rest of the cat's life. Other options were kidney transplant and dialysis, as in people. Some people elected the option of putting the cat to sleep. I discussed these options with Karen. She paused, and then requested me to give the cat the first fluid therapy. She decided not to take fluid bags for continued therapy at home. I knew one time fluid therapy would not be enough to help a cat with renal insufficiency. However, I thought that Karen needed a chance to think about her cat's future over the following few days, considering the cat's age.

I saw Karen again a week later and I asked her about the cat. She said, "The cat is doing fine, eating, drinking well, playful, and acts like a brand new kitten." I smiled and asked, "What did you do for the cat?" She said, "I prayed for her." Her answer instantly penetrated the fibers of my soul. My smile immediately vanished and I stared at Karen, and the harsh memories and the crying voice of my son and his sufferings and my prayers suddenly came into view as a live show.

Without any hesitation, I said with a begging and quivering voice, "Karen, may I ask you for a favor? Would you please pray for my son?" She replied positively, "Yes." She asked me for his name as well as what medical problem he had and I told her. A week later on September 1, 2000, I received an unexpected phone call from Karen asking about my son's health status. I had almost forgotten about my conversation with Karen about my son. I said "Nothing new. He is still on the same medications." She raised her voice as if annoyed and said, "Stop all the medications. Your son is cured. Good bye." She hung up on me.

I was puzzled for a minute while I stared at the phone handle. Although I considered myself a true believer, I wondered "What is this? Has G-d finally sent me an angel in form of Karen to tell me that my son is cured or what?" Any bombshell — even a sweet one — required time to digest. I went into deep thought for a minute. I decided to listen to the messages of these three incidents and to Karen in particular. After all, I was the one who started the conversation with the Almighty G-d and I requested Him not to leave me alone in deciding on the fate of my son's gut. Apparently a spark of faith was kindled and turned the path of my thinking upside down. I felt that I was receiving Divine corroboration. I went home after work and suggested to my wife to reduce Sam's medication dosage and to see what would happen. She agreed with me. The most toxic of all medications that my son was taking was cyclosporine. He was taking 100 mg twice a day. So we reduced the dose to 75 mg twice a day, starting September 1, 2000, as the first step.

Our visits with Dr. M. were scheduled every month for a routine checkup and to discuss results of his blood work. A few days prior to the visit, we usually went to the laboratory for blood work. The results were available to Dr. M. upon our visit. September 7, 2000 was our next scheduled visit with Dr.

M. In that visit, Dr. M. started by saying "Sam's blood values were excellent. They were never like this before." His sedimentation rate, a blood test to measure intensity of inflammation was normal and so was his hemoglobin, a test for anemia.

To say the least, I was amused to hear Dr. M.'s good news, as if I took the full credit for it. I felt overjoyed for the first time in a long time. I leaned back in the chair I was sitting in, crossed my arms behind my head, and cleared my throat before I asked Dr. M., "What is his sedimentation rate now? What was it in the past?" She said, "It is 5 (normal is 0-15) now, and in the past it was always high in the range of 95 to 100". She asked me with a smile, "What did you do?" She knew I was a veterinarian and that I was trying anything desperately to cure my son. I said to Dr. M. "I talked to Him," while pointing my finger up to the sky. She giggled, but maintained her stare at me waiting for another answer. I smiled because it crossed my mind that Dr. M. might think I was going crazy considering how much I was involved with my son's issue. When she heard no other answer from me, she gave up and said, "Well, continue doing whatever you started. It is working."

Sure enough, we continued to reduce the dose of cyclosporine. As of October 7, 2000, Sam was not receiving cyclosporine at all after taking it twice a day for two and a half years. We were so encouraged because his blood values remained excellent in subsequent tests. Cyclosporine was the most valuable medication to control my son's illness and keep it in remission. We continued to do what we started which was gradually taking Sam off his other medications, one after another.

On October 24, 2000, there was only one medication left out of six that my son was taking. It was the prednisone. It felt so great that we could stop giving these toxic medications to my son, and that surgery is no longer needed. Sam was cured. He continued to do very well. This was due to a series of unexplainable events and the stories of three women during a very critical time when we had to decide whether to do surgery or not. Thanks to You G-d.

We started to taper the prednisone very slowly and gradually on October 24, 2000. We were having fun doing this. Blood values remained excellent during November 2000 and early December 2000 as well. Sam had no inflammation, his sedimentation rate was normal, his anemia was gone and his hematocrit was 45, which was the highest ever in his life so far. We were so happy that Sam was not taking any of the other medications and that he was now only on a half dose of the prednisone, which was about 5 mg a day. Dr. M. was very curious about what was I doing with my son to get these wonderful results.

CHAPTER 4

The Final Destination

SAM'S PATH TO SURGERY:

For almost 4 months, we had been tapering the medications Sam was taking. His health appeared at its best and we were so very happy. Unfortunately, our happiness did not last for long. On December 21, 2000, Sam started bleeding again. To say we were only deeply saddened was unjust to our horrible feelings. Blood values started to reverse in a bad direction. We had no choice but to put him back again on a full dose of cyclosporine and prednisone to stop the bleeding.

On January 11, 2001, Dr. M. recommended surgery again. She commented "no medication would cure his problem. If he was my son, I would have done the surgery a long time ago." Sam's friends at school were teasing him about being short and hairy, which upset him and made him cry. Dr. M. said that he will never grow in height while being on a high dose of prednisone. My wife became convinced about the surgery and started to question my refusal to consent to the surgery.

I was confused at this point. I thought G-d had sent me two women to deter me from surgery and had sent a third woman to stop the medication. I had followed His messages. Now, I did not know what to do. Under the circumstances of lack of response to medications, the toxic effects of these medications, the social challenges and teasing of my son by other children, the strong recommendations of Dr. M. the physician, and the questioning of my wife, I gave up. I felt cornered from all directions. I started unwillingly leaning toward surgery.

Why Was I Reluctant To Accept The Surgical Option?

I was very reluctant to consent to my son's surgery for various reasons. Fact number one is that once they cut his colon, it is gone forever. Fact number two is that the medical approach to treat ulcerative colitis was getting brighter every day. New medications that targeted and inhibited enzymes, proteins, and cells that were involved in the inflammatory activity in ulcerative colitis were being tested at that time. New drugs were being introduced all the time and were increasingly successful. I was optimistic and hoped for a new wave of UC treatments that would control his illness without surgery. Fact number three is that doctors were not absolutely sure whether Sam had Crohn's disease or ulcerative colitis. Sam had many overlapping features of both diseases. At times, it sounded as if he had both diseases at the same time racing in his gut. It has been reported in the literature that it can be extremely difficult to distinguish between these two diseases. Several tests were performed on my son to tell these two diseases apart. Unfortunately, the tests were inconclusive. As a matter of fact, the blood test that was used to tell these two diseases apart was negative. In other words, Sam had neither ulcerative colitis nor Crohn's disease. As I mentioned before, the test was repeated three times while he was under the care of doctors in Alabama, Delaware, and California. Also the test may give negative results under certain circumstances such as if the disease was in remission.

Findings in tissue samples examined under the microscope suggested that Sam had ulcerative colitis but did not definitely rule out Crohn's disease. Some suspicion remained overcasting the diagnosis of my son's illness.

The need to differentiate between ulcerative colitis and Crohn's disease was fundamentally essential in order to make a decision about surgery. In UC the inflammation was limited to the large intestine, and therefore surgical removal of the large intestine was considered a "cure" of ulcerative colitis. Whereas in Crohn's disease, the inflammation may affect any part of the gastrointestinal tract from the mouth to the anus, therefore surgical removal of the large intestine as planned for my son would not be a cure of his illness if it turned out to be Crohn's disease. Crohn's disease could recur after surgery in the remaining parts of the digestive tract. Crohn's disease had been confirmed in patients thought originally to be suffering from UC. In spite of advances in research and diagnostic tests, doctors were still having difficulty in a small proportion of cases differentiating Crohn's disease from UC and my son was one of them.

STRAIGHT TALK WITH THE SURGEON:

Dr. M. referred us to meet Dr. D.P., a surgeon in Northern California. On February 1, 2001, we visited Dr. D.P. He was a very impressive and talented surgeon. Dr. D.P. was one of a few in the world who pioneered a surgical technique for the treatment of ulcerative colitis. In 1971, he was the first surgeon to place an internal pouch in patients with UC. His technique was adopted around the world. He was a world renowned surgeon who lectured all over the world about his surgical techniques for the treatment of UC. Wow, what more could one ask for in a surgeon?

"You have no choice but surgery. I have never seen a patient on so many medications for so long," Dr. D.P. commented in our meeting. He added that Sam was short primarily due to the colitis rather than the prednisone. He will grow in height quickly once his toxic colon was removed from his body. He would do much better in school and would have a better quality of life without his diseased colon. His message was very strong saying, "Don't leave the room without consent to surgery."

Dr. D.P. described in detail the surgical procedure for us with drawings and diagrams, and patiently answered all of our questions. He would remove the entire large intestine and join the small intestine either to the groin area or directly to the anus, depending on health condition of the anus and whether ulcers, fissures or cracks were present on the lining of the anus. He would make this decision based on these findings while Sam was on the surgical table and not at anytime prior to that. These fissures or small cuts or tears in the anal canal were commonly found in persons with UC. They were painful and they often bleed and because of their location they made it very painful to have a bowel movement.

Dr. D.P. added that Sam would stay in the hospital for seven to ten days and that it would take six to twelve weeks for him to retain control of his bowel movement. He would have soft stools for the rest of his life. Finally, he discussed possible complications of the surgery which are basically the same for any surgical procedure.

We asked Dr. D.P. at the start of our meeting whether Sam needed to be present. Dr. D.P. firmly said, "Yes. I want him to listen and to trust me." Sam was with us in the room and listened to the entire discussion without expressing any negative signs, concerns, or emotions. Sam was only 6 days away from his 7th birthday on February 7. Dr. D.P. gave me a bunch of his publications on his surgical techniques to read at home. He also handed me a list of patients on which he had performed his surgery with their phone numbers and addresses so that we could contact them if we desired.

SAM WAS ADMITTED FOR SURGERY:

We tried to taper the dose of prednisone prior to the surgery based on doctor recommendations because it could delay healing after surgery. However, Sam flared up once the medication dose was lowered. On March 9, 2001, we called Dr. D.P. to schedule the surgery as early as possible.

On March 29, 2001, Sam was hospitalized for pre-surgical testing and a clean-out. An intravenous catheter was placed in his arm to give him fluids and a tube was inserted through his nose to the stomach. In addition, he was given enemas to clean up his bowel in preparation for surgery.

The morning of March 30, 2001 was Sam's surgery day. He was 7 years old. His weight was 59 pounds and his height was 43 inches, which was the same as it had been for more than 4 years. During the first two years of his life, he was in the 90th percentile for height and now at the 10th percentile.

The anesthesiologist and his team came in first to the pre-anesthetic room around the surgical suite and explained to Sam the procedure of anesthesia. Sam turned his face and offered me a smile. The anesthesiologist was wondering what was all that about. My wife explained to them that Sam had been watching his dad, who was a veterinarian, administer anesthesia during surgery on dogs and cats. The anesthesiologist was excited to hear that Sam was very familiar, not only with the anesthesia procedure, but with the pre-anesthetic medications and gas maintenance anesthesia as well.

I was standing beside Sam's bed facing him and holding his hand with his mom when he was given the pre-anesthetic medication and kissed him good bye at 11:41a.m. Sam was very brave as usual. He remained very calm. He never cried or expressed any signs of fear or emotion. Nurses, assistants, and doctors were amazed by his courage and incredible bravery. He had never been afraid, mad, angry, or fearful of anything. He had a great insight to what going on with him.

When the nurse started pushing his bed away toward the surgical suite, Sam turned his face towards me and stared at my face with a calm expression as if he thought this was his last time he would see me. I felt that our souls communicated at that moment and exchanged love to each other without saying a single word. I sensed him saying, "Dad, I love you, in case I do not see you again." I controlled myself so hard not to cry in front of him. He maintained that fixed stare at my face until the swinging doors of the surgery area were closed. Immediately, my tears started flowing uncontrollably. These were very emotional moments.

Counting The Minutes, While Our Son Was On The Surgery Table

Sam came out of the surgical room at 5:22.p.m. of March 30, 2001. That was 5 hours and 41 minutes. My wife, our daughter, and I were sitting in the waiting room the whole time and counted the minutes. The anesthesiologist came out first and told us the good news. The surgery went very well and Dr. D.P. did a very nice job. An epidural line was inserted in Sam's back to drip pain control medication for two days following surgery. Then, Dr. D.P. came out and gave us even better news. It was one step surgery. The entire colon was removed and the end of small intestine was directly connected to the anus, so there was no hole in the abdomen and no external pouch.

I had the opportunity of looking at his colon. There was not a single spot of a normal looking colon. The entire colon was extremely damaged. The walls of the colon were greatly thickened and appeared red-blue with prominent blood vessels. Ulcers were present all over its lining. The colon appeared angry and scary. The doctor explained that Sam's colon was in danger of perforating, which was a potentially life threatening situation. Although I was glad to hear about the successful surgery, at the same time I was so frightened to imagine what my little boy went through.

Dr. D.P. was very excited about the procedure and both my wife and I were excited because of his confidence and the good news. He added that no blood transfusion was needed even though we had two units ready for him just in case. Finally, Dr. D.P. said Sam had a lot of little black seeds in his intestine. "What does he eat?" We all laughed. The little black seeds were the Pentasa medication. Once the Pentasa capsule is broken in his stomach, thousands of little black seeds are freed out. We had always seen these seeds in his stool. "The only thing you will be sorry for is that you did not consent to the surgery earlier," Dr. D.P. said before he said good-bye to us.

The surgical procedure was called the j-pouch surgery. In Sam's case, it involved the removal of the entire large intestine (colon, rectum, and appendix) at its junction with the small intestine. Then a loop of the last four inches of the small intestine was surgically modified to form a sac or pouch to act as a reservoir for stool, and the end of the reservoir was attached to the anus. Most of the web tissue holding the intestine together was cut to stretch the small intestine. The small intestine was held to the remaining surrounding tissue by surgical metal staples that we could see every time they took X-rays of Sam's abdomen.

At 7: 26 p.m. of March 30, 2001, Sam opened his eyes in the recovery room to see me standing next to his bed. I offered him a smile but he was still in another world. Gradually, but slowly, he woke up fully from the anesthesia and was back to himself by the following morning.

He had made excellent progress within a short period after surgery. Sam started walking on the second day after surgery. He started eating solid food while still in the hospital. He no longer needed medication. The prednisone was tapered very slowly after surgery to give a chance for his body to take over and start producing steroids normally.

He was discharged from the hospital 10 days later, on April 9, 2001. The night of discharge, he had his favorite Chinese food for dinner. In the morning, I heard Sam sneak from his room to go downstairs by himself. Later, I realized that he had eaten the left-over Chinese food for breakfast. I thanked G-d for everything.

CHAPTER 5

Adjusting To Life Without A Colon

FOLLOWING SURGERY AND DISCONTINUING OF medications, Sam appeared more healthy, active, and playful right away. He started to grow noticeably in both height and weight. Sam had been on steroids for years. Impaired utilization of calcium occurred as a side effect of prednisone. Steroids also tended to decrease the number of bone-forming cells in the body. This may have contributed to Sam's poor growth, in addition to the effects of his very bad ulcerative colitis. During the first year following surgery, Sam grew 5 inches taller and gained 4 pounds. The bad side effects of the medications started to disappear gradually as well. He no longer had a moon face or a hairy face and hairy arms. Sam's young age, good general health, and his positive attitude helped him to recover rather quickly from the surgery. The surgery was a tremendous gift that greatly alleviated the physical pain my son had felt daily. Life after surgery was different than life with a sick colon and it was definitely worth it.

Date	Height in inches	Weight in pounds
Feb 7, 1994	21	8 (day was born)
Mar 5, 1995	34	25
Oct 30, 1996	43	38 (start of ulcerative colitis)
Sep 7, 1997	43	43
Oct 1, 1998	43	47
Oct 7, 1999	43	49
Sep 30, 2000	43	55
Mar 30, 2001	43	59 (day of surgery)
Apr 18, 2002	48	63
April 9, 2003	52	75
Jul 28, 2004	55	95
May 3, 2005	56	111
Dec 1, 2006	61	133
Dec 1, 2007	62	140
Dec 1, 2008	65	160
Feb 17, 2009	68	171
Aug 30, 2010	68	165
Apr 19, 2011	68	165
Apr 30, 2012	70	172
Mar 1, 2013	70	176
Mar 1, 2014	70	179
Mar 30, 2015	71	175

SURGERY AFTER CARE:
Routine checking of Sam's pouch was performed once or twice a year during the years following surgery. This checkup was done under general anesthesia with one day of hospitalization. In this procedure, the pouch was irrigated and cleansed and samples of inside of the pouch were taken for examination under the microscope. Occasionally, Dr. M. used the opportunity of Sam being under anesthesia to scope his esophagus, stomach, and small intestine as well for monitoring purposes. She may also have taken tissue samples of the various scoped parts for the same reason.

His routine laboratory blood tests values were normal except for mild anemia. Although no blood could be seen in his stool, he seemed to be losing very tiny drops consistently. No source of bleeding could be detected on endoscopic examination. However, very tiny blood spots could be undetected. He also continued to take iron daily.

On the day of surgery, Sam's large intestine was sent in its entirety to a specialist for his opinion. The specialist concluded that the slow bowel movement that Sam had was secondary to the inflammation rather than primary nerve damage. They also raised a concern based on features seen in these tissues that Crohn's disease could not be entirely excluded, although no definitive evidence of Crohn's disease was seen.

Post Surgical Complications:

Although Sam was doing great following surgery, his health was not completely free of complications. He had fecal incontinence and leakage, dehydration, pouchitis, fistula, and abdominal adhesions.

1. Fecal incontinence or lack of control of bowel movement
   How bad is the leakage?

   Fecal incontinence was a serious problem that faced Sam for almost five years after surgery. Soreness and itching of the skin around the buttocks area was caused by the leaked stool.

   The reason for the liquid stool was water exceeding the ability of the remaining small intestine to absorb. The main function of the small intestine is absorption of nutrients from the food we eat. The main job of the colon was to absorb water. Following surgery, Sam no longer had a colon. Therefore, his small intestine had to carry out all functions of both the small and large intestine. The small intestine needed to absorb not only the nutrients, but the water as well, and to act as a reservoir for the stool. This was an overload that the small intestine was not used to. The small intestine needed time to get used to carrying out these additional functions. Sam had to go to the bathroom more often but his chance of getting colon cancer was drastically reduced.

The leakage continued day and night and was most frequent immediately after surgery. It gradually decreased in frequency and became sporadic years after that. Leakage stopped completely approximately five years after surgery.

2. Dehydration
   How serious is the dehydration? What contributes to the dehydration? What are the signs of dehydration? How can dehydration be prevented and treated?

   Dehydration was another serious problem due to Sam's water loss in stool, leakage, sweating from physical assertion and not drinking enough. Dehydration is dangerous for anyone and certainly more so for young patients with ulcerative colitis.

   The body needed a certain amount of fluid and electrolytes to function properly. Once signs of dehydration appeared on Sam, such as sunken eyes, dry mouth, dark circles under eyes, sleeping more often with lack of energy, complaint of abdominal pain, loss of appetite, and reduced urine output, only aggressive intravenous fluid administration will correct his condition. In other words, oral intake of fluids would not correct his dehydration regardless of how much he drank.

To compensate for electrolytes lost in stool, Sam regularly drank liquids rich in electrolytes such as Gatorade. He also took salt tablets to encourage drinking and consumed vitamins/mineral supplement.

Advanced symptoms of dehydration included abdominal pain and occasional vomiting. The pain was unmanageable on occasions without hospitalization and aggressive fluid therapy and pain medications. The first of these dehydration episodes started about two months after surgery on May 24, 2001. On that day, Sam started having severe abdominal pain, excessive vomiting, and stopped eating. He was hospitalized at 11:00 p.m. that evening with suspicion of obstruction in the small intestine. Sam responded well to fluid therapy and antibiotics intravenously and was discharged five days later.

Sam exhibited these episodes of dehydration very frequently during the first year following the surgery. It began to get less frequent as time went on. He was hospitalized 13 times for these episodes on May 24,

2001, June 4, 2001, January 21, 2002, May 22, 2002, June 24, 2002, August 10 2002, August 25, 2002, September 18, 2002, March 12, 2003, May 12, 2003, August 4, 2004, May 3, 2005 and September 19, 2006. Each hospital stay lasted approximately five days.

Dehydration was the primary cause of the pain episodes leading to the sluggish bowel motility with subsequent accumulation of gas and fluid within the intestine. On abdominal radiographs, the gut appeared distended with gas and fluid as if it was obstructed. Sam seemed to respond rather quickly once he was rehydrated without further efforts. To get him rehydrated he often needed several bags of intravenous fluids.

Most of these hospitalizations were during the first year after surgery, when the small intestines were still adapting to taking over the extra load of water absorption. Also, most of these hospitalizations were during the warm months of the year in California, which further implicated the dehydration's role in his pain episodes. Once Sam was rehydrated, he became himself again with no pain. He was very active and regained his normal appetite.

During these hospitalizations, he would undergo extensive blood testing, radiographs with and without barium, urine and stool tests, and occasionally endoscopic examinations of his esophagus, stomach, small intestine, and the pouch. In almost all of these hospitalizations, the findings were unremarkable and Sam would suddenly improve once he was well re-hydrated.

3. Pouchitis
   How to prevent pouchitis?

   The pouch was created using Sam's small intestine to act like a rectum to hold stool until it was expelled in the usual fashion. On March 12, 2003, Sam was hospitalized again for dehydration and vomiting. He responded well to aggressive intravenous fluids and antibiotics. This time, ulcers were seen on lining of the pouch. Examination of tissue samples were taken from the lining of the pouch and revealed features of pouchitis (inflammation of the pouch).

   This was the first time pouchitis was confirmed by laboratory tests. Pouchitis occurred again once a year for four years until 2007. The exact cause of pouchitis was unknown but pouchitis is common in post-surgical patients with ulcerative colitis. Pouchitis is treated with antibiotics. Probiotics intake may help prevent pouchitis.

4. Intestinal fistulas
   What are fistulas and how to recognize them?

Another complication of ulcerative colitis and more so in patients with Crohn's disease was the fistula formation (tunnel-like passage between two adjacent structures). This occurred when intestinal ulcers progress deep through full thickness of the bowel wall forming a tract. These tracts may connect the intestine or pouch to the lumens of adjacent organs such as the bladder or to the outside of skin. When a fistula opened in the abdominal cavity it leads to the escape of waste into the abdomen, causing severe abdominal pain and fever. Intestinal fistulas that connect to the skin may drain blood, pus and stool through the skin.

In early June 2004, Sam started to complain of low grade abdominal pain, which continued intermittently for weeks. He was seen by Dr. M. and was diagnosed with pouchitis. Flagyl and Ciprofloxacin antibiotic medications were not very effective this time.

The pain was intensified. On August 4, 2004, Sam was admitted to the emergency hospital for severe abdominal pain and vomiting. Numerous blood and stool tests, as well radiographs of the abdomen did not reveal unusual findings. Urine tests revealed the presence of bacteria that normally were found in stool. Doctors started to suspect a fistula between the urinary bladder and the pouch.

An exploratory abdominal surgery was performed. During this procedure, numerous adhesions were seen between loops of the intestine and between the intestine and the urinary bladder. Another adhesion area was noted between his urinary bladder and the pouch. After the adhesions were freed up, a fistula was identified between the pouch and the urinary bladder and was corrected. The surgery lasted for three hours. Sam was discharged after 21 days of hospital stay.

5. Adhesions
   Why do adhesions happen and how do I know I have them?

Abdominal adhesions between loops of the intestine were due to scar tissue build up, which occurred commonly following abdominal surgery. These adhesions pulled loops of the intestine in opposite directions like ropes resulting in tightening and narrowing of the lumen of intestine. When excessive, the surrounding scar tissue could cause pressure narrowing or blocking of the bowel and interfere with proper movement of the intestine.

Symptoms of intestinal obstruction included severe abdominal pain, vomiting, cramping, severe bloating, and the inability to pass gas. Intestinal obstruction may also result from the thickening of the intestinal wall caused by the excessive inflammation and scarring.

6. Narrowing of anal sphincter
   From constant diarrhea to the difficulty of pooping

   Sam was hospitalized on May 3, 2005, because of the narrowing (stenosis) of the anal canal. This was caused by the scar tissue formation and tightening of the canal. He complained about the difficulty to defecate. It was corrected surgically under general anesthesia.

7. Pouch ulcerations
   How to fix them?

   During the hospitalization in 2005, a small ulcer was also noted on lining of the pouch which was excised and corrected.

Starting in 2007, 6 years after surgery, Sam appeared to be free from these complications, except for the loose stool, which we understood would continue for the rest of his life. However, he appeared to have good control of his bowel movements with no more leakage. He drank a lot of fluids. His last hospitalization was in summer of 2007 for the routine checkup of the pouch.

THE EMOTIONAL IMPACT OF ULCERATIVE COLITIS:

Chronic illnesses are dealt with in different ways. Some families appeared to have little emotional reaction, while others experienced a great emotional strain. This was because a chronic disease poses a threat to person's well-being and feeling of security most. Young children had a different set of concerns when they were ill. However, their parents or caregivers would definitely have another set. Any disease could seriously impact your way of life if you allowed it. This did not mean we should ignore diseases in our systems, yet too much worrying did not help cure the illness either.

A. EMOTIONAL IMPACT OF ULCERATIVE COLITIS ON SAM'S LIFE BEFORE SURGERY

Sam was under 3 years old when his illness started. He did not know the impact or nature of his illness, other than the unpleasant and frequent bouts of diarrhea, abdominal pain, and cramping that bothered and upset him. He also did not know the side effects of the medications he was taking every day, yet he hated to take them regardless. Gradually, he got very frustrated taking several medications two to three times every day as he did not understand how important it was to take them. Some of his medications tasted awful.

The misery associated ulcerative colitis symptoms. Sudden and unpredictable diarrhea attacks in public were not uncommon in patients with UC and this was a big fear for any human being. It was very embarrassing, dignity challenging, and awkward to defecate in your pants. Bathroom accessibility and the ability to clean up after the attack were real concerns facing patients with UC, not to mention not making it to the bathroom on time. Anyone who has UC could attest to the misery associated with this illness. Sam needed to have immediate access to a bathroom because holding it in was not an option. UC was a miserable nasty disease that could control your life and degrade you.

Sam suffered from diarrhea for more than 5 years prior to surgery and leakage of watery stool for another 5 years following surgery. Drops of waste may leak every few minutes. Wet spots on his pants and the smell of stool were hard to hide from other people and were hurtful, especially among children who did not understand what Sam was going through.

The daily constant social challenges: At 5 ½ years of age, Sam started going to kindergarten. He also started to express interests in things like karate, musical lessons, bicycling and etc.

Being in public, he started to face social challenges from other kids.

Sam hardly grew an inch for 5 years while he was suffering from ulcerative colitis. He also had hair overgrowth on his body and a puffed up face because of some of the medications. Kids teased him and said "Why are you short?" and "How come you have mustache?" Kids in school could be innocently cruel in such circumstances.

Sam became very sensitive to their comments. They had certainly hurt his feelings and his self-esteem. He started to get irritated and angry rather easily. One day, he told his mom, "I cannot control my bad behavior with my sister. It is the kids picking on me, Mom. It is not because of the medicine." Weeks after Sam joined karate, his friend joined karate, as well. But his friend was placed at a level higher than Sam. Sam learned that he was initially placed at a lower level because he was short.

Easing schooling with ulcerative colitis: Sam had frequent flare ups and several hospitalizations which caused him to miss a lot of school. In such circumstances, it was difficult to strike the right balance between maintaining privacy and revealing enough to get the support and help Sam needed from his teachers. His chronic absences made it hard to keep his illness from his teachers, friends, and classmates. Letting them know even minor details seemed to help Sam share his feelings with his close friends.

The school nurse and teachers were made aware of his illness and he was able to get permission to leave the classroom often without asking every time, either to visit the bathroom or to get his medication from the school nurse. Additionally, teachers were helping him catch up on make-up work and material. They fully understood and accepted his extended absences due to the flare ups and hospitalizations.

Easing travelling with ulcerative colitis: In California, we lived close to San Francisco and we used to go out almost every weekend to Fisherman's Wharf, China Town, and Golden Gate Park to have some fun time. Keeping Sam busy seemed to distract him from his illness. However, it was not uncommon to notice him lagging behind us while walking and seeing him tightly crossing his legs to hold a sudden attack of diarrhea or having intense facial expressions of painful straining.

At the beginning of his illness, we always carried extra diapers, our own toilet paper, and hand sanitizer when we went out. At a later age, our top question was finding the nearest bathroom. In addition we carried extra underwear and additional zip lock plastic bags to store the old pair. Ulcerative colitis was a nasty disease that allowed your bowels to control your life. It was a big deal to go anywhere, because you did not know when you needed to go the bathroom next.

Having a positive attitude helps. Prior to surgery, and while in remission, Sam was involved in various activities almost on daily basis. Kids seemed to deal with issues as they arise. They did not dwell on what they had or overthought about its future impact and consequences. They cried when they had a flare up and played when in remission, without linking the two situations together.

In spite of all of the miseries associated with ulcerative colitis flare ups and the frequent hospitalizations and daily medications, the disease did not seem to have caused Sam any serious emotional reaction. He remained very social, wanted to go to school, and participated in various activities. He participated in physical education and sports with his classmates as much as he could. On days when he did not feel well or couldn't run, he said so, and sat down or just walked. He expressed interest in wrestling and started to practice with his colleagues after school. He was not shy to express his feelings.

II. Sam's life following surgery

Sam continued his positive journey to a good life following the surgery. He had a huge abdominal scar from his two major surgeries, but this did not prevent him from swimming in public and in front of other people. He had a great sense of humor, which sustained him throughout the tough times in his illness. He was always smiling, laughing, and joking, so it was impossible not to like him. He could fit in any situation comfortably.

Sam did not have to take medications following his surgery. This fact, coupled with the disappearance of the residual side effects of his medications, like hairy body and the puffy face, were big plusses to up lift his mood. Moreover, Sam started to grow in both weight and height remarkably soon after surgery, and his body proportions started to appear like a healthy boy.

Impact of fecal leakage on Sam's daily life and activities following surgery: Sam continued to leak watery stool for 5 years after surgery. The rash and soreness on his buttocks caused by the leakage were so painful that on occasion, they prevented him from going out to play or even to walk.

In addition to applying skin lotion and rash cream, Sam used to take several showers throughout the day to wash away the leaked stool and to help relieve the pain caused by the rash. Night showers were taken on hourly intervals for months after the surgery. This had greatly disturbed his sleep and intensified his fatigue. Not to mention, this disturbed the sleep of his family and had an impact on our performance the next day. I admit I was very reluctant to get up at night during a relaxing sleep. Consider the impact of getting up five, six or seven times a night to take a shower on a seven year old boy. Sam became so exhausted due to the frequent showering at night that he occasionally fell asleep while standing in the tub taking his showers.

One day he shouted "*I hate my life. This surgery messed up my life.*" I became so emotional, sad, and sorry to hear that my seven year old boy made such a strong statement.

Does positive attitude help? Although Sam suffered from ulcerative colitis at young age, he never let his illness stop him from enjoying his life. His optimistic outlook of life may, in part, have helped him to cope well with his illness. He continued to lead a playful and enjoyable life even though he occasionally needed to take medications for pouchitis and was hospitalized.

He enjoyed his daily activities as much as he could. He rode his bicycle and scooter almost all of the time with his friends. When he turned ten, he developed an interest in motorcycles, and he got a pocket bike when he was eleven. Then, at age twelve, he developed an interest in ATV'S and dirt bikes. We visited sand dunes in various places and he was as adventurous as we all knew him to be. He jumped off high hills and drove fast down steep slopes and had a lot of fun. At age eighteen,

Sam got his first car, and at age twenty, he got a motorcycle. Now, we hardly see him at home, except at nights.

The learning curve and coping with flares: Over time, it appeared that Sam had learned that his "illness" would be with him for a while and that his soft stool would be with him for the rest of his life. He appeared to have accepted this fact realistically, without self-pity, without guilty-feelings, and without blaming others for his illness.

Dependency and care giving: Although at an early age, Sam showed some dependency on me or his mother, in terms of self-reliance, he became gradually independent and he became more self-sufficient as he got older.

In addition to the pain and suffering from his illness, Sam also experienced much more in his hospital stays. He met so many nurses and doctors, received so many IV's and shots, and had so many medications and tests. This helped him gain maturity at a very early age. Currently, he socializes with older friends, rather than people his age. He appeared to value life more than his peers. He liked to play games and to gain the experience of older kids.

Ulcerative colitis did not interfere with Sam's success in life. Although he missed so many school days, he caught up with his classmates in school and achieved high scores. Basically, his illness did not affect him academically, in spite of missing school for weeks on occasions. He was never held back in school.

At grade 8, Sam became a member of the school's wrestling team. He participated in competitions with teams from other schools and won his very first wrestling match. He was talented, strong, and full of youth. As parents, who had for a long time watched their child ravaged by his colitis, we see him today athletic and we are thankful and proud.

In 2012, Sam graduated from high school, received his driver license, and a car. In February 2014, he graduated as a medical assistant from a local college. He enjoyed his job serving patients and paying it forward to his community. Now, he seemed to be more concerned about other sick children.

The memories of ulcerative colitis miseries are history. At the time I wrote this book for publication in 2015, Sam was 21 years old. I mentioned to him his early illness; the pain, sufferings, and frequent hospitalizations. Surprisingly he knew that he was sick and that he had surgery because of the huge scars he had on his stomach, but did not remember anything else besides that. Although his illness had left a huge scar in my memory, I felt so thankful that all he remembered of his illness was a scar on his stomach. I was glad that all of the brutal memories, sufferings, and relapses were not apparently retained in his memory, or at least they did not seem to affect his current life at all.

III. Emotional impact of ulcerative colitis on the family

A chronic illness within a loved one was never good news. Patients and their caregivers felt like there was an ominous cloud hanging over their lives. This cloud could take a toll on all aspects of their lives and there was always the threat of a flare up. The impact could be felt on many levels: physically, emotionally, socially, economically, and spiritually. Chronic illness could leave one and his family with a profound sense of devastation.

How can ulcerative colitis emotionally influence parents? Chronic illness in a child could cause parents to become overprotective, and the illness could become a source of tension and frustration in the family. In particular, parents might become alarmed when their child lost weight, ate poorly, became anemic, and had frequent bouts of diarrhea, or the warning signs of potential emergency. This was an addition to the worries of administering medication on time, avoiding triggers, and assuring the child was having a happy time.

On top of all this, parents had to take care of their personal daily affairs, as well as to take care of other members of the family. For caregivers, the stress associated with ulcerative colitis in their loved one could feel like a double whammy. On occasion, it was very tough to balance all of these issues.

One of the hardest parts of caring for my child was watching him while he experienced pain. This was beyond any words I could find to describe my feelings and emotional devastation. We moved to four states in less than three years to look for the doctor who could cure our son. This young child was hospitalized twenty six times, had general anesthesia twenty three times, had endoscopic examination twenty one times, several radiographs and CT scans, had two major surgeries averaged of four and a half hours each, had five blood transfusions, and countless doctor visits. We stayed with him in the hospitals for so long that the hospitals felt almost like our home.

The emotional and mental health effects of our son's illness had impacted us as a family from the start. We soon realized that we were dealing with a disease that was out of control and has no cure. It was an unpredictable illness. There was always the threat that the disease may flare up at any day and at any time with no prior notice. It could flare up at night, early in the morning just after you woke up, on the way to go to work, on the bus to work, while you were in a business meeting, on family's first day of planned vacation, on your birthday, on the first day of a new job, at the grocery store, or in an airplane.

No one could guess when remission could be attained, or for how long it would stay. Patients and their caregivers needed to learn to deal with uncertainty. It was very difficult to live a normal life with the threat of ulcerative colitis flare hanging over our heads. Frequent, unpredicted flare ups and hospitalizations could wreak havoc on a family plan and daily life. We had to abruptly cancel plans and changed our life style. Bad UC, like what my son had, could literally rule someone's life and their families. It impacted my son and my family in almost every area of our lives for years including work and leisure. It inevitably changed our family dynamic. The constant need to use the bathroom definitely affected his daily activities.

While staying with my son in the hospital, I forgot to take care of myself on certain days, or get enough rest or exercise. To have a decent meal in a relaxed environment or at least a well-balanced diet other than fast food became wishful thinking while being far away from home. In addition, there was the emotion of missing my other family members, friends, and work.

It seemed that regardless of how much I trained myself on how to deal with stressful situations, and regardless of my high level of stress tolerance, I failed to avoid feeling burnout on occasions. For four years, I endured what some might call hell.

Do parents feel self-guilt? When we were asked "any other member of the family on either side has this disease?" it is impossible not to feel the implication that we might somehow be responsible for the sickness of our child. In addition to all of the painful emotions, the parental guilt feeling never left me alone. Did I cause this to happen to my son? Was it my genetics? Did I trigger his illness somehow? We felt so sorry our son had to suffer so much. Instead of enjoying his childhood playing with other kids in the neighborhood, he spent his early years of life sufferings in hospitals. We shared years of our son's illness, anger, frustration, and grief.

Caregiver knowledge helps: My training also helped us understand what our son was going through. I searched the disease extensively and became very aware of my son's illness. I kept extensive daily notes on his symptoms, response to medications, diaries of his food he was eating, description of his pain and its level, activity level, laboratory reports, and recognizing his potential warning signs of a flare up to quickly get him under control.

Also, to learn about the disease helped a lot in seeking support from the right places. I frequently called doctors and other healthcare professionals with questions and was always in contact with the Crohn's & Colitis Foundation of America for information. Luckily, I also had a high tolerance for stress and stayed upbeat throughout the years of his illness, for most of the time.

Recognize symptoms of depression and seek professional help early: Regardless of how medically knowledgeable and stress tolerant the patient and their caregivers were, they would feel the stress and perhaps some degree of depression at one point or another. Depression affects energy levels tremendously. Depressed people feel fatigued, less motivated to do work, and less interested in things they used to enjoy. As a result, such people become less punctual at work than they used to be, and may have a hard time to finish their tasks and responsibilities. Students became less interested in finishing homework and their grades slip. Depressed people tended to isolate themselves, became less interested in making plans with friends, did not return calls or attend social activities. Seek professional help as soon as you notice a loved one with any of these symptoms. This would be the key to return to a normal functioning and enjoyable life.

Try to change the family focus of attention: About one month after surgery, I brought home an orange Tabby male kitten. I thought this might do the trick to change the tense atmosphere at home. The entire family immediately fell in love with him. He was very playful and funny. He changed everyone's feelings for the best. Sam was so excited and immediately bonded with the kitten. It was his first pet. He named him

Habibi, which means "my love" in Arabic. The kitten started to sleep with Sam every night. The kitten became a new focus of attention and changed the mood of the whole family.

How to manage the potential high costs of ulcerative colitis treatment without going broke? The cost of living with UC could be considerable. There are financial responsibilities to copay medical bills, hospitalizations, prescription medications, laboratory tests, and follow up care. My son had two major surgeries that cost more than a hundred thousand dollars each. He had to be hospitalized several times before and after surgery, which cost tens of thousands of dollars each stay. The cost of routine blood and stool tests, doctor visits, X-rays, colonoscopy, etc. could drain any budget. Even with a good health insurance plan, the member still had co-payments and plan deductibles.

In addition, I had the responsibility to support and care for the rest of my family. Frequent absences from work, leaving jobs, moving out of state, trying to find a new job, and loss of income in between were additional financial burdens. In our first move, we had to sell our house in a rush.

The Crohn's & Colitis Foundation Web site had links to programs that could help with payment of prescribed drugs, copays, and related care. Buying generic medications rather than brand names could help as well. Finally, if your condition kept you from going to work or doing things you want to do, you could apply for disability benefits from Social Security.

Planning our future following surgery: Soon after my son's surgery on March 30, 2001 Sam's quality of life improved right away. His illness became less disturbing to our life and daily activities. We no longer had to plan to locate a nearby bathroom. I started to see the light at the end of the tunnel. I felt that our incredible story was approaching its final chapter. I sensed that the painful years were behind us and we were about to settle for good. We all felt like we started our life again in March 30, 2001, the day of the surgery.

The medical bills mounted and the waves of stress we had been going through for the past four years seemed to have reached their peak and started to descend. What a great way to move forward with life. I started planning for our future. The first step I thought about would be to open my own veterinarian hospital to promote my income instead of working for others. I took out a loan and established my own hospital in northern California.

In February 2002, I announced the grand opening of my hospital. My wife helped me in the morning while the children were in school. Sam helped me sometimes in the afternoon after school and on weekends. The hospital was doing fantastically well right from start. I worked really hard and I was able to become debt free within 2 years.

Chronic illness and residual stress can shred the family. Unfortunately, our happiness did not last for long, in spite of having a healthy child once again and a new business. My wife and I got separated within 6 months after I opened the hospital, and then we got divorced some 6 months later. The children lived with their mom at first. Two years after my divorce, I sold the hospital, moved out of the area and settled in Southern California. G-d responded to my prayers and both of my children followed me and lived with me. I felt that life started to sprout back again in my body. I became alive once again and in a better mood. I decided to have a new fresh start. So I built another veterinarian hospital near Los Angeles and happily started working on my own once again.

Sam had been my assistant when not in school and my daughter helped me during the summer holiday break. Health-wise, Sam had been doing great with no hospitalization or pain episodes since 2007.

Last but not least, the kitten "Habibi" that boosted our mood was now 14 years old. He was becoming an old man, was less active, and had a deep voice, but remained healthy.

How To Choose The Right Doctor For Your Loved One With Ulcerative Colitis

It is worth mentioning that what I experienced and learned from visiting so many doctors and traveling from one state to another regarding how to choose the right doctor.

Normally, your primary care physician would refer you to a local specialist (gastroenterologist). However, not all gastroenterologists were equal. Some had more experience than others in certain areas. Some might have deal with patients suffering from UC on a daily basis, whereas others may see a patient with UC once a year or two. Some were experienced with UC in children, like doctors in children's hospitals, while others had experience with the UC in young adults. Some doctors had extra training and interest for example in liver diseases, while others specialized in inflammatory bowel disorders. Some doctors were involved in research on UC and were aware of new treatments and diagnostic tools. Some doctors were board certified by the American Board of Internal Medicine which meant they had met strict requirements for training and had passed a rigorous examination in their specialty. Some hospitals had treatment centers devoted to UC and Crohn's disease that offered more cutting edge therapies. You needed a gastroenterologist who was experienced with UC.

We searched for the best possible health care provider for our loved one. We selected a gastroenterologist who treated patients with UC on regular basis, who had current knowledge on the disease, and whom we felt comfortable with and could trust.

Resources other than our primary care physician helped us find the best. Resources included our health insurance company, Crohn's & Colitis Foundation of America, Crohn's & Colitis Advocate Group, Web sites, other patients with colitis, local medical schools, and Children hospitals.

Crohn's & Colitis Foundation of America
386 Park Avenue South, 17th Floor
New York, NY 10016
Phone: 1–800–932–2423
Internet: www.ccfa.org

United Ostomy Associations of America
P.O. Box 512
Northfield, MN 55057–0512
Phone: 1–800–826–0826
Internet: www.ostomy.org

Crohn's & Colitis Advocate Program
Phone: 1-888-857-0634
www.crohnsandcolitisinfo.com/Advocate-Program

Did G-D Respond To My Prayers?

I continued to pray to G-d to heal all sick people. I was certain that G-d would never break his promise "*call upon me and I shall respond.*" Unfortunately, Sam underwent surgery and lost his colon. I did not think surgery was what G-d wanted for Sam. G-d could have healed my son without surgery. Certainly, G-d had a reason and purpose in all of this. He created people when they were unmentioned. Sure He was able to fix their defects. My patience was tested repeatedly by G-d. I thought I passed, maybe not with flying colors, but passed nevertheless. I may have failed on a couple of choices when I lost it while watching my son suffering. That was when I felt I lost all my strength and hope and hit rock bottom. I was wrong. I never gave up hope from the Almighty G-d when tragedy struck. Instead, I prayed to G-d to strengthen my faith in order to understand what my loved one was going through. I believed that everything happened according to G-d's will and was for the best of our interest, even though it appeared otherwise.

In July 2008, Sam and I travelled to the Holy lands in Israel and Saudi Arabia. We prayed at the sacred places like in Jerusalem and Beth Le-hem. Then we went to Saudi Arabia and prayed at the sacred House of G-d in Mecca that was founded by the father of all prophets Abraham and his son, Ishmael. Since these visits Sam had not been hospitalized or had complained from any issue related to his ulcerative colitis or the surgery to this day of writing this book in 2015. Was it a coincidence? I did not believe so.

In 2010, which was two years after our visit to Israel, I developed interest in going to a local temple to learn about Judaism and started reading the Torah for first time in my life. I was amazed one day to read the following verses in "The Second of Chronicles" in the "Old Testament." In the grand opening ceremony of the House of G-d in Jerusalem, which was built by Prophet Solomon, the Prophet kneeled upon his knees and spread his palms out to the heavens and started to pray in front of all the congregation of Israel. Prophet Solomon listed among his requests the following verses **6:32** *"And also to the foreigner who is no part of your people Israel and who actually comes from a distant land by reason of your great name and your strong hand and your stretched-out arm, and they actually come and pray toward this house,* ***6:33*** *then may you yourself listen from the heavens, from your established place of dwelling, and you must do according to all for which the foreigner calls to you; in order that all the peoples of the earth may know your name and may fear you the same as your people Israel do, and may know that your name has been called upon this house that I have built.*

I continued to read with great attention that G-d Almighty had responded positively to prayers of Solomon: **7:12** *G-d now appeared to Solomon during the night and said to him: "I have* *heard your prayer, and I have chosen this place for myself as a house of sacrifice.* **7:15** *Now, my own eyes will prove to be opened and my ears attentive to prayer at this place.*

In his prayers, Prophet Solomon requested G-d to respond favorably to people who pray at His house. The Prophet provided detailed descriptions of those people to include foreigners like me and my son. Both my son and I were Americans and we were no part of the people of Israel. We were not Jewish. We travelled from a long distant land, the USA, to Israel and prayed toward His Great Name. I thanked Prophet Solomon for his prayers and above all I thanked G-d Almighty who listened to our prayers at His house and ended the sufferings of my child and stop the heart wrenching feelings that his family went through.

We thanked all people who prayed for my son. We also thanked all doctors and nurses who took good care of Sam.

I prayed to G-d that sharing our story with others could support those out there who were going through this terrible illness and who suffered both physically, emotionally, and spiritually. Amen.

Did you enjoy this book?

If so, please donate to Crohn's & Colitis Foundation of America (CCFA).

The CCFA is counting on your financial support to advance life-changing research for Crohn's disease and Ulcerative Colitis. Although significant progress in understanding these diseases have been made—there's still much work to be done. Through your donation, we can continue to fund all of our vital programs.

Your generous tax-deductible gift will help fund critical research for improving treatment and finding cures for all inflammatory bowel diseases. It will also help sustain support programs for those who are struggling with the physical and emotional toll of living with Crohn's disease and ulcerative colitis.

Here are ways you can support the Crohn's & Ulcerative Colitis Research financially:

Donate online
Make a gift in honor of someone or in memory of a loved one
Commemorate weddings, birthdays, or other special occasions
Leave a legacy through planned giving
Multiply your gift's impact through an employer match
Transfer your stock
Donate your vehicle
Join Take Steps
Participate in Team Challenge
Create a personalized fundraising page

Please visit the CCFA website and select your method of contribution: www.ccfa.org
Select explore CCFA Research and then Support CCFA Research.

CCFA, 733 Third Avenue, Suite 510, New York, NY 10017
800-932-2423

Index

Apriso medication for ulcerative colitis, 38

www.ingramcontent.com/pod-product-compliance
Lightning Source LLC
Chambersburg PA
CBHW021424170526
45164CB00001B/80
* 9 7 8 1 5 0 0 2 7 8 9 6 0 *